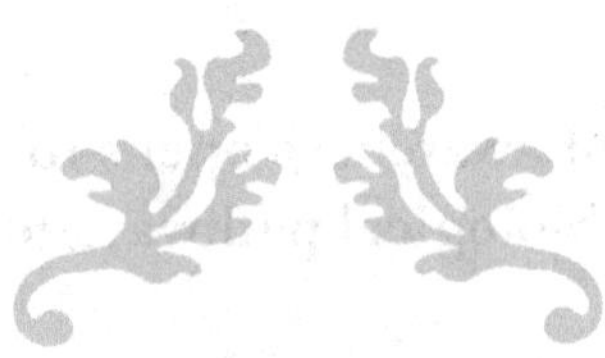

---

# Perceiving Wellness Beyond Limitations

---

## A Higher Perspective on Healing Clinicians and the Healthcare Delivery System

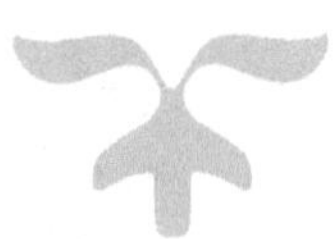

Darnell Osburn, RN, BSN

Legal Nurse Consultant

Reiki Master

**About the Cover:**


**The light of awareness opens to a cognizance,
allowing biological pathways to respond.**

# Dedication

This book is dedicated to all healthcare brethren who are enduring any dimension of suffering. May the words and concepts within this text generate the energy to view every situation from the highest perspective.

**"Our greatest weakness lies in giving up.** The most certain way to succeed is always to try just one more time." ~ **Thomas Edison**

**"Although the world is full of suffering, it is also full of the overcoming of it."** ~ Helen Keller

# Contents

# Preface

"To a large extent, whether you suffer depends on how you respond to a given situation." ~ Dalai Lama

**"The natural healing force within each of us is the greatest force in getting well."** ~ Hippocrates

**"Make every effort to change things you do not like. If you cannot make a change, change the way you have been thinking. You might find a new solution."** ~ Maya Angelou

**"Imagination is more important than knowledge." "The important thing is not to stop questioning. Curiosity has its own reason for existing."** ~ Albert Einstein

"Why did this happen to me?" This question asked by too many of my patients highlights the physical and emotional burdens of receiving a diagnosis of a chronic disease. Adjusting to a new incurable medical condition and the odds of survival evoke an awareness of life's unpredictability and uncertainty of the future. While some patients have accepted the limitations of their healthcare system, others are evolving in their perspectives. An increasing number of medical consumers believe that conventional medicine frequently overlooks natural therapeutic options that could enhance their health. By understanding why patients seek healing outside their healthcare system, providers can effectively assess and address their patients' needs and preferences.

Ethical concerns arise when patients perceive their medical system placing efficiency (temporary relief or symptom management) over avoidable suffering by not investing in root-cause based medicine. Therefore, this text represents a concerted effort to fully understand the genesis of chronic diseases so their causes, not their effects may be addressed. This text invites each clinician to participate in addressing important issues in care through collaborative and proactive problem-solving approaches. It does not advocate for rejecting modern medicine; instead, it calls for its broadened application. Healing transcends simply following standard protocols; it involves understanding the unique individual behind the illness. This understanding helps to pinpoint the factors contributing to chronic disease. By addressing all disease constituents, healthcare providers can create a more personalized treatment plan that resonates with each patient's needs and preferences. Identifying underlying causes encourages a holistic approach that views patients as multidimensional individuals, rather than mere cases to be managed under the disease-based model. Considering this shift promotes a deeper connection between healthcare providers and the individuals they serve, cultivating a more compassionate healthcare system.

Patients want to understand and address the underlying causes of their conditions for sustainable health outcomes, rather than having to forever manage their symptoms. Many of my patients believed that more comprehensive therapies were available despite being told by their providers that chronic conditions were irreversible. Some point to disparate transparent biomedical research findings, *reversal of some chronic diseases at lifestyle centers, and those who have experienced spontaneous remissions (chapter 8).

Cutting-edge research articles and patient inquiries can be examined from a broader perspective** to support advancements in medical practice and enhance practitioners' understanding of complex medical conditions. Intrinsic motivational processes (Di Domenico & Ryan, 2017) may help identify a conceptual model of disease (chapter 6) that shapes clinical trials (chapter 3) aimed at enhancing the identification of root causes, therapeutics, and prevention strategies. The medical community's commitments to these insights could have been better timed to help my sister. Barbara, who suffered from a chronic disease, was consistently told by her providers that healing was impossible, and she would have to live with a permanent medical condition. Furthermore, they predicted her condition would only continue to deteriorate. Were they right, or did their authoritative assertions, presented as fact, infiltrate not only her beliefs but also those of our family? Thus, did events unfold as a result of aligning with each practitioners' expectations (the nocebo effect). (Colloca, 2023)?

In the mid-1970s, a sense of medical idealism inspired me to pursue a career in nursing. I believed that becoming a nurse would enable me to enhance the lives of my sister and all my future patients. My first role as a charge nurse in a psychiatric hospital allowed me to witness the challenges individuals faced while coping with a mental illness and many times, a physical condition. Subsequently, I met a nurse case manager who hired me as a staff nurse in another notable New York hospital.

In the coronary intensive care unit (CICU) there, I experienced a dichotomy between witnessing my sister endure a chronic medical condition and striving to heal the sick. At that time, physical and psychological factors were not always considered as interconnected; therefore, patients' symptoms were frequently treated separately. When symptoms are addressed in isolation, underlying issues can go unrecognized, potentially leading to incomplete or ineffective care. While working in the CICU, a clinical drug trial affected the perceptions and realities of patients and staff when unintended effects of the experimental drug occurred. My experiences in both hospitals deepened my understanding of the complex relationship between emotional and physical health (chapter 6).

During this decade, experiments advancing the theory of neurotransmitters modulating memory with chemicals became accepted. Clinicians, still reeling from the findings of cellular memory research studies from the 1960s, struggled to comprehend the newly published accounts of near-death experiences. Then on its heels reports of people experiencing spontaneous remissions.

Despite the documentation provided by licensed physicians, medical communities dismissed instant healings reported by individuals who had experienced life beyond their fixed perceptions as fabricated, embellished, or impossible.

Discrediting these firsthand witnesses undermined prioritizing scientific investigations into credible accounts of how these instantaneous healings occurred. These enigmatic testimonies, deemed far from the threshold of reality, could never establish a new standard for healing. Or could these encounters be viewed as catalysts for deeper inquiry to broaden awareness of existing human capabilities (chapter 8)?

Providers interpreting symptoms originating from external factors or internal malfunctions on its face, depreciated mind-body synergism as influencing biological functioning. Then, why did some individuals address experience wholeness by utilizing non-traditional methods? As these types of government studies are currently underway (chapter 5), medical professionals can accurately assess (chapter 3) the evolution of revisions or indistinguishable recommendations.

This text presents biomedical researchers' perspectives on the etiology of disease expressed as symptoms to appropriately address human suffering. Before her passing, Barbara had posed her own existential questions. She often questioned why she had to endure years of suffering, finding it unfair that life could be so challenging, even cruel at times. Like many patients, she could not reconcile her pain and suffering with any meaning or purpose. The term "suffering" holds certain personal and collective significance, creating the foundation of truth experienced as reality. While working in intensive care units, medical professionals often saw suffering as a form of distress that sometimes escalated to torment, despair, and even death. It was as if pain and suffering disrupted any possibility of inner peace, while mortality offered an escape from these constant burdens. As nurses, our core mission to patients was centered on the commitment of alleviating any form of distress causing suffering. Many patients seeking relief from suffering view it as a fundamental right and an obligation of their medical providers and healthcare system.

Over the years, each personal and professional experience of human suffering yielded the same inquiries. "What factors lead to suffering, and if it is not an essential aspect of existence, how can the research sector and medical community identify its underlying causes and provide permanent relief?" "Is accepting patient suffering consistent with medical ethics?" This posture activated a series of inspirational events. I enrolled in another university and graduated with a Bachelor of Science Degree in Nursing. Decades later, after learning about a complementary medical approach, my interest in energy led me to become a Reiki Master. My curiosity about nonconventional and ubiquitous medical systems continued to heighten. The spirit of inquiry intensified with each nursing role. As a nurse case manager, I attempted to assist patients seeking relief from the symptoms of their chronic disease(s), which their healthcare provider advised was unavailable. Many other events spurred a decade of extensive research that complemented past and more recent scientific investigations, leading to shared conclusions. These papers highlighting gaps in existing knowledge, increased my awareness of many valuable and transparent findings.

Having completed their own investigative and healing journey, some healthcare providers have taken conscious steps toward full client service. This faction of licensed doctors, psychologists, and practitioners* representing higher patient expectations is perceived as operating outside the perimeter of conventional medicine. For decades, these providers have been conducting research and providing a human-centered whole-care approach in their private practices, holistic, and lifestyle care centers. The public's clamor for health freedoms has fueled the creation and sustainability of such wellness clinics. Some of these constitutive physicians have challenged mainstream norms by lobbying their government legislatures. However, their scientific experiments supporting the utilization of successful multilayered healing approaches were not considered viable for comprehensive integration into an established healthcare system. Can medical care confidently advance within the consistency of the same framework?

Have vexations within the current healthcare structure inspired the readiness to confront them? Unpacking complex concerns prompts universal questions. "Are most healthcare providers and medical consumers content with the fulfillment of their medical system?" "If exceptions exist, what are the next conscionable steps?" "Can a medical system expediently assess itself, identify, strategize, and apply revisions to fully address the complexity of chronic disease?" "Does the recognition of relieving existential distress imply health as a human right, thus, a national obligation?" If so, then this right can be seen as extending to people accessing a more precise medical product. Do clinicians believe they are experts in self-care to impeccably lead by example? If this were consistently so, medical professionals worldwide would be caring for their charges free of the symptoms reflecting unresolved root causes. Chronic sensations often require clinicians to live and work in distraction and discomfort.

So, how can clinicians transcend overarching mainstays to become the vanguard of healthcare advancement? The foundation of this strength advances through impeccable biomedical scientific practices (chapter 3) and perceiving beyond collective limitations creating a space for broader perspectives. Limitations derived from clinicians' former education and experience can support perceiving inevitable diagnostic destinies. The collective medical perspective accepts that everyone will eventually fight against predetermined fates or surrender to their predictable paths. These beliefs grounded in the reality of linear thinking have become the only logical, rational, and traditional view; any discordance disputes the confines of accepted reality.

Furthermore, these concepts prompt insurance companies to acknowledge and compensate for diagnoses and services considered normal, predictable, and, consequently, reasonable and customary. Do these standard terms adequately reflect fidelity and justice to insurance payers and their subscribers?

That is, have medical systems been open to diverse scientific findings supporting the providers* who are already successfully practicing them? Some issues noted in current practice involve prognostication, which has been based more on experience and the element of ***chance. New levels of awareness of specific disease determinants and prospective interventions (chapter 6) based on scientific investigators' studies bear further evaluation. Can a healthcare system ever imagine providing patients with the blueprint for healing chronic disease? The answer to this question determines its reality.

This text raises questions and concerns many biomedical researchers, healthcare professionals, and medical consumers share. It presents researchers' conclusions that may differ from one's personal or professional beliefs, prompting curiosity in diverse research areas and analytical thought. Open-mindedness generates interest in negotiating universal challenges. Clinicians choosing to perceive beyond current standards prevent continuing any ineffective habitual practices.

In nursing practice, my friend never accepted the status quo. Since "Annie" was a Registered Nurse, her physician believing her disease-specific symptoms were imagined justified sending her home. After a second opinion, relief of an ovarian cancer diagnosis started a fear-based life as anxiety about her fate escalated. Post hysterectomy, she wondered if standard protocols would fulfill their intended function. Eventually, inadequate responses to shared decisions led to the most difficult choice. Could this confrontation have been avoided by perceiving this human as a whole being? If her symptoms were psychogenic, would a complete workup concurrent with a mental health consultation have generated a correct diagnosis and potentially a different outcome?

This error in misdiagnosis may appear to be an isolated incident. However, this one human being was part of nearly 12 million affected by misdiagnosis annually in the United States (Singh et al., 2014). These statistics reflecting a stark gap in healthcare delivery bear an immediate response. Should we dismiss this concern as honest mistakes? Acknowledging millions of diagnostic errors that result in no treatment or inappropriate therapy (chapter 5) serves as a catalyst for identifying the root cause of this systemic issue. Unlike an impartial coin toss, assessing symptoms involves estimations that may be biased and violate the probability threshold. *** (Arkes et al., 2022). "78.1% of physicians overestimated the combined probability of 2 events compared with the probability calculated from their own estimates of the individual events, leading to mathematical diagnostic and prognostic error." (Arkes et al., 2022).

Professional duty and fundamental human protections in averting preventable harm have mobilized an organization. In 2021, the Society to Improve Diagnosis in Medicine initiated a strategic plan to improve correct diagnosing (chapter 5). However, in 2019, "Annie" could no longer continue nonfunctional interventions and slowly transitioned. She became a statistic, one among the millions that year who encountered a deficiency in clinical expertise. Could her tragic trajectory have been prevented? If her providers had viewed this situation from a broader or higher perspective** (without emotions, judgments, or preconceived opinions) they may have created a path of possibilities and the opportunity for a different outcome.

Presenting concerns about care is not an appeal to oppose pharmaceuticals, the medical community, or any specific medical specialty. These institutions possess distinct qualities that contribute to their value. Contextual questions raise the need for a movement and a call to action aimed at restoring both professional and public confidence in the medical product. Otherwise, consumers may continue seeking relief from their suffering elsewhere. How do you perceive assessing your healthcare system's efficacy: as irrelevant, an opportunity, or improvement as an impossibility? There are significant barriers hindering medical care advancement. One is the issue of academic gatekeeping.  Many researchers and organizations won't grant permission for citations of their completed research articles. This restriction can be seen as a lack of transparency that limits the accessibility, assessment, evaluation, and potential dissemination of valuable information. Consequently, these limitations hinder the integration of current knowledge.

The following obstacles are relevant across all areas of practice. Between 2016 and 2019, the period from "Annie's" diagnosis to her passing, scientific journal articles discussing a cadre of researchers' concerns were available. While "Annie" and her medical providers could have accessed these articles online during that time, many researchers and organizations currently do not allow their papers to be referenced. This reluctance may stem from various concerns; however, such restrictions hinder access to vital information that could assist current providers and patients in making well-informed decisions regarding therapies.

Many researchers have expressed concerns about conflicts of interest (COI) influencing the recommendations and guidance of oncology guideline authors based on insufficient evidence. This level of professional concern typically lays the foundation for requiring more substantial evidence to address potential ethical issues. During this period, compensation to oncologists may have limited transparency and accountability (Open Payments program, cms.gov). Although some journals include addressing COI to promote transparency, all medical journals can consistently use this practice. (Teixeira da Silva et al., 2019).

A confluence of researchers challenging the foundation of medical practice are attempting to preserve the evidence-based medicine archetype. They are calling for the reconciliation of disparities to uphold the cornerstone of medical output: quality care and patient satisfaction. Naturopathic doctors and integrative medical physicians generally focus on identifying the origin of disease, thus prioritizing cures over merely managing symptoms. Will the medical community's awareness of consumer expectations align with supportive research findings to adapt care strategies? Providing healthcare services with persistent delivery challenges direct the medical system's responsibility to investigate all issues and options. By fully acknowledging and addressing known industry concerns, practitioners can better avoid harm and legal repercussions.

Objectivity without preconceived answers inclines a higher perspective** that expands potential within the known unknown and the unknown unknown. Curiosity and openness advance the therapeutic potential of the medical profession. Clinicians who perceive beyond collective limitations activate a dimension of personal authority and professional command. Providers who comprehend underlying causes of disease are better equipped to heal themselves and, ultimately, those they serve. Existing within an expanded perspective on healing prompts considering the full spectrum of the human condition in wholeness, wellness maintenance, and prevention measures.

While some practitioners may welcome assessing and evaluating their current healthcare system, others may feel uncomfortable. Is the existing framework the sole viable option thus, necessitating the status quo? A different perspective encourages critical discussions within the medical community about root-cause-based medicine, ultimately enhancing care and medical consumer satisfaction. Perception's filtering of this content and the forthcoming information shapes personal reality (chapter 2).

# Introduction

"The art of medicine consists of amusing the patient while nature cures the disease." ~ Voltaire

"The physician treats with words; within the physician-patient social system, the patient is moved by fears and other sentiments, and these are modified by the physician's words and phrases. Physicians dispense not only medicines but words that influence medicines or, all by themselves, that affect the patient more than the medicine." ~ Dr. Morgan Martin

"If the brain expects that a treatment will work, it sends healing chemicals into the bloodstream, which facilitates that. That's why the placebo effect is so powerful for every type of healing. And the opposite is equally true and equally powerful: When the brain expects that a therapy will not work, it doesn't. It's called the "nocebo" effect."
~ Bruce Lipton

Is it possible that my friend's death could have been prevented? This thought weighs heavily on my mind, as I reflect on the moments leading up to that tragic day. To me, "Annie's" passing signified the loss of an incredible friend and nurse. Had the medical system failed her, or did this one human being have to rely on overcoming its imperfections? In 2016, the delayed diagnosis of ovarian cancer (with subsequent metastasis) created an urgent timeline for evaluating and choosing therapies. Was there full awareness of everything she was about to place complete confidence in? Through the lens of a patient, a specialized medical team implied the prompt transition from illness to wellness. This belief negated the need to evaluate her providers' perceptions of peer concerns (Preface) regarding the then-standard interventions. Did selective collective provider perceptions hinder awareness of research data that might have soon become mainstream?

There was a wealth of research information on cancer available from 2016, the time of her diagnosis, to the end of her ordeal in 2019. During that time, research indicated that the cellular foundation of geometry influences homeostasis and biological organization, and that cells can reorganize in the opposite manner. The predictability of metastasis is based on cancer cell morphology. (Lyons et al., 2016). Early detection of the physical characteristics and appearances of cancer cells to determine aggressiveness of the cancer was not immediately clear due to a delay in diagnosing. In 2015, researchers at the Mayo Clinic Cancer Center in Florida discovered that restoring normal microRNA (miRNA) levels in cancer cells could reverse abnormal cell growth. (Anastasiadis, 2015). Immunotherapy (Koury et al., 2018) and Right to Try legislation (United States (U.S.), 2018), which permits terminally ill individuals to access eligible experimental therapies (chapter 1), were available but not considered. Complementary medicine for cancer patients, as described on some U.S. government websites, was deemed impractical.

Was a dissonance in the perception of professional heuristics (a trial-and-error approach) and patient expectations (timely relief of suffering by cure) accountable for my friend's demise? The agony and despair my friend experienced reached the depths of my being as she slowly wasted away. Can the medical community foresee a way to prevent such suffering from recurring, or will medicine continue to perceive illness in the same manner? Can medical systems that excel in acute care overcome their current limitations to improve treatment options for individuals suffering from chronic conditions? Is a healthcare system that offers preventative, and healing measures obligated to address well-known issues? If so, will medical systems focus on the foundational practices (research, chapter 3) that underpin the identification of the antecedents of diseases to treat them from their point of origin? If a healthcare system fails to do so, can it lead to legal repercussions (chapter 9)?

As beautiful "Annie's" life hinged on continuing measures generating unintended effects, time was of the essence. If patients are not being perceived as identical to others in the same circumstance, then what factors create a discrepancy in response to the same therapeutic stimuli (chapters 3 & 8)? As well as cancer cells evading apoptosis, researchers have found that the nocebo effect (Preface) can influence patients and their sentient cells. As cells have a consciousness (Baluška et al., 2021), they analyze and react to their environment accordingly. These findings suggest that negative expectations can potentially lead to real physiological changes, highlighting the powerful connection between the mind and body. Then, understanding the nocebo effect may play a crucial role in enhancing patient care and outcomes.

Did my friend's cells learn to analyze and respond to the synergistic meaning of words declared by those in authority, evoking pessimistic thoughts and emotions? "Each and every tiny cell in our body is perfectly and absolutely *aware* of our thoughts, feelings and of course, our beliefs." (Rao et al., 2009). "Belief-reinforced awareness becomes our biochemistry." (Rao et al., 2009). Many researchers have discovered that, like advanced algorithms, cells can be programmed, navigate through layers of language, and interpret their environments, thereby shaping their perceptions and actions (chapter 6). Since my friend interpreted the statement, "There is nothing else we can do," as evidence of truth and fate, perhaps she experienced the unintended effects of her prescribed interventions and gave up. As "Annie" expected a cure, what was the difference between her outcome and the documented cancer survivors' spontaneous remissions? If investigation into the diagnosed terminally ill and then cured (chapter 8) guides medicine into the uncomfortable, the unexplainable will always be fearfully archived.

As the worldwide public awaits answers to these confrontations, many are seeking solutions elsewhere. Despite the lack of scientific community endorsement, patient perspectives of current healthcare delivery have been a driver in the pursuit of a better way. Can mere awareness of the ability to counteract authoritative opinions (chapters 1, 2, & 8) influence patient outcomes?

Researchers have found there is power in words spoken by those in authority. Words that evoke feelings of limitation, hopelessness, and helplessness can significantly impact individuals if they perceive and internalize them as their truth (chapter 2). "Adverse nocebo responses can cause harm to patients and interfere with treatment adherence and effects in both clinical practice and clinical trials." (Colloca, 2023). Would a different outcome have emerged if the previously unsinkable "Annie" had never accepted or integrated another's definitive limiting statements as indisputable truths? Many individuals see themselves as victims of their circumstances, but could they, in fact, be casualties of someone else's decisive beliefs?

Someone in authority presenting their strong beliefs or predictions as hardened, undeniable facts raises the question of whether it's possible to challenge them. It suggests a tension between subjective certainty and objective reality in discussions about medical prophecy. Did the situation prompt my friend to imagine and create a scenario to fit another's perception of reality (chapters 2 & 8)? Could mere perceptions, phraseology, and scientific curiosity have prevented human suffering? Ultimately, this issue raises deeper philosophical inquiries about the nature of belief and one's truth (chapter 2).

As a final effort, would her provider's research on the documentation of others' spontaneous cancer remissions contradict the established medical canon? The exploration of these extraordinary cases (chapter 8) promotes a more open-minded approach to causal mechanisms and potential treatment options (chapter 6), encouraging further investigation into the mind-body connection and holistic healing practices.

The purpose of highlighting my friend's journey is not to disparage any specific therapy, medical system, or provider. Instead, it creates an opportunity to enhance the medical product. Some may view a healthcare system that ignores the call for higher performance as showing indifference or malfeasance (chapter 9). Blame was not assigned to my friend's providers, who offered, devised, and delivered conventional treatment plans. However, what is the medical community's response to the current and future chronic condition sufferers expecting a different experience? In both research and clinical settings, diverse questions without preconceived expectations increase the likelihood of discovering alternate answers.

Healthcare professionals were among those experiencing traumatic stress and illness during the 2020 pandemic. As this suffering continued into 2021, the top-trending Internet searches became "how to heal," "mental health," and "affirmations." Believing that something beyond conventional methods exists, many individuals with chronic conditions continue seeking medical resources online.

As lifestyle medicine providers successfully reverse some chronic illnesses, will researchers become more interested in building upon their scientific findings to enhance the predictability of outcomes? Chronicling the challenges and successes of both professional and patient experiences better informs future care perspectives (chapter 9). Clinicians aware of persistent issues affecting care practices bear the responsibility of confronting and resolving them (chapter 5). Only through a commitment to address current challenges can a sustainable healthcare system that meets the needs of providers and medical consumers be created. Attention to patient concerns strengthens the medical community and promotes public trust. Fundamental science and open science practices enhance objectivity, aiding the shift from the abstract to the tangible.

# Chapter 1

## The Conundrum of Health

"The more we see health as a practice rather than as a problem to fix, the more we encourage the body's natural potential to be healthy." ~ Aarti Patel

**"If you want to find the secrets of the universe, think in terms of energy, frequency, and vibration." ~ Nikola Tesla**

**"Whether you think you can, or you think you can't - you're right." ~ Henry Ford**

**"Replace judgement with curiosity." ~ Lynn Nottage**

The infectious disease doctor's notes had just sealed her fate. The proof was in the biomarkers indicating sepsis. This laboratory result would forecast another's inevitable surrender. Everyone predicted that multimorbidity and compromised immune system defenses would yield to a new bodily insult. Each provider note implied my newly assigned charge would eventually decline and leave the intensive care unit (ICU) via the morgue. However, the provider's prognosis did not align with my patient's understanding of the circumstance. Despite acknowledging the potential of intravenous vancomycin to combat methicillin-resistant Staphylococcus aureus (MRSA), she asserted her own therapeutic approach. This patient's personal beliefs made our first encounter a memorable one.

While donning required personal protective equipment (PPE) outside my patient's isolation room, all staff behind the nurses' station stared intensely. Their facial expressions seemed cautionary. "Was this an indication that more vigilance was required before entering?" "Oh, what a silly thought; how could this ICU room be any different from the others?" Nevertheless, the question persisted. "What was behind this door?" Once inside, the energy was quite different from the fast-paced environment of just a moment ago. There was a sense of peace as a small blonde-haired woman looked up.

While smiling, this patient's compression-stocking feet dangled over the side of the hospital bed. After introducing myself, she said, "Welcome." Seated, her medium-framed, dark-haired spouse nodded in agreement with her every word.

Then, in the very next moment, it was as if they suddenly appeared. Countless stones and crystals of all shapes, sizes, and colors adorned what was considered final accommodations. The patient's eyes remained fixed on me as she revealed her palms to the multitude of stones. My eyes and ears remained fully alert as she drew a deep breath and parted her lips. With the highest personal authority, it was declared, "These crystals will heal me!" A profound silence followed. Were the staff's non-verbal signals finally understood, or would there be further convictions pushing me beyond my comfort zone?

My patient's words and the way they were delivered sank in as I was doffing my PPE. Could these utterances reflecting personal intent really shape one's desired future? At the nurses' station, everyone negated this patient's deep conviction of restoration and stood with the agreed-upon odds. The medical team doubted that vain mitigation efforts could ever overcome her desired trajectory. When another person's reality doesn't align with ours, challenges can arise. Staff silently dismissed this person's belief in stones as their hands sporting diamonds and gemstones cared for her and their wrists relied on crystal technology (page 3). While this compromised patient and their medical team saw things differently, each remained steadfast in their beliefs. Can a clinician's perception open or collapse the space to favor one potential or another? This common unintentional practice may hold the space for life or death as substantiated by the power of negative conditioning (below). It is known that people may experience side effects or worsening due to staff expectations of treatments and outcomes. Verbal suggestions, prior experiences and observing others experiencing adverse effects can trigger the nocebo effect. (Colloca, 2023). Clinicians assuming specific results as evidence of fate may impact those susceptible to influence (Chapter 2). However, this patient continued to live with a level of awareness or understanding that deepened her connection to a personal desire. When faced with adversarial updates, she refused to accept another's interpretation of reality, which contradicted her own certainty.

One day we learned that my former patient was being discharged from a step-down unit. It was gratifying to know she defied staff expectations and would leave the hospital just as she entered. Was this a profound lesson to this ICU staff in underestimating one's beliefs, will, and power to create? Everyone agreed the unexpected had occurred; however, curiosity ended there. However, what was the driving force behind making the previously unthinkable possible? Can people naturally encode their DNA to effectuate healing (Chapters 2, 7, & 8)? A primitive movie of a racehorse was encoded in bacteria DNA and successfully replayed. (NIH, 2017). Dr. Leonard Zon explores the function of a "don't eat me" signal and identifies a possible therapeutic target using cellular barcoding and single-cell RNA sequencing to potentially treat leukemia. (Zon, 2023). Is encoding living human cells to store specific information the path forward?

Some believe an intentional focus energizes natural encoding Therefore, they consciously direct their constant inner dialogue to intentionally influence biological functioning. Some perceive gemstones as possessing a vibrational frequency (energy) that connects to the crystalline grid, promoting healing. Quartz, tourmaline, topaz, and garnet can exhibit a piezoelectric effect and convert mechanical vibration (energy) into electrical energy. (Qian et al., 2020). As a result, they find application in diagnostics and various medical devices that utilize crystal technology. "Piezoelectric nanoparticles exposed to ultrasonic waves can change the viability of breast cancer cells." (Zaszczyńska et al., 2020). "Piezoelectricity enables certain materials to generate an electric field in response to mechanical deformation." (Kao et al., 2019). Are perspectives on the healing aspects of crystals like thoughts and prayers that align with a specific vibrational energy (Chapter 8)? The energy of repetitive thoughts is powerful as they become beliefs and create personal reality. "Beliefs become a reality as this level of awareness integrates into one's biochemistry." (Rao et al., 2009). Cell biologist and scientific researcher Dr. Bruce Lipton, Ph.D., says that that the brain will manifest the picture we hold, which can be overridden by creating a new program. (Lipton, 2024). Many believe that cancer only holds a genetic component. Cancer is not heritable but aligns with epigenetic changes that alter gene expression. (Aydin & Kalkan, 2020).

Emotional turmoil from judgments, anger, resentment, and shame moving through a being may activate cells into a state of conflict (Chapter 6). While people don't always overtly display negative emotions, they may be suppressing them. My former patient seemed focused on the appreciable effects of medical care and the power exercised by personal beliefs.

At the time, comprehensive complementary and alternative medicine (CAM) practice standards did not exist. While tolerance for their usage existed, open-mindedness about them did not. The staff continued to view this patient with subtle judgment, attributing their eventual recovery solely to the efforts of conventional medicine. Many medical professionals generally attribute healing without mainstream medicine's involvement to the placebo effect. This patient may have experienced a different outcome, as verbally and nonverbally, there was a potential for staff to unwittingly advance the nocebo effect. (Hansen & Zech, 2019). That is, one or more people may have integrated their beliefs into another's biochemistry. (Rao et al., 2009). Everyone dismissed CAM practices during my patient's admission, hospitalization, and discharge as they considered this patient an aberration, an exception to the rule, and an outlier. Can medicine advance by investigating such medical contradictions (Chapter 8)?

Decades ago, CAM practices were considered foreign, unscientific, and downright crazy. Although some still consider them as such, in the United States, 38.3% of adults and 11.8% of children use some type of CAM therapy. (CDC, 2007). The World Health Organization (WHO) estimates that 88% of all countries use traditional medicine, indigenous, or other treatments; thus, data is being sought to establish frameworks and standards for them. (WHO, 2022). In the meantime, in the face of a person's unwavering faith, belief, and survival instinct, can healthcare professionals advocate mutually giving up? Practitioners believe they are advising of the reality of predictable outcomes and prohibit providing false hope. The false hope harms argument promotes protecting providers from people who have been diagnosed as terminal from making unreasonable requests for help. To support medical ethics (Chapter 5), can medical opinion collaborate with one's autonomy?

Hope acts as a driving force, motivating individuals to pursue their goals. Some providers opine that by offering or acknowledging hope to anyone they deem incurable is unrealistic and drains healthcare resources. However, CAM interventions such as guided imagery, crystals, supplements, and energy practices don't involve healthcare utility but are generally handled as out-of-pocket expenses. Prayer and optimism, offering different perspectives and vibrations, are free. Hopefulness aligns with a vibratory state leading to the excitement of the prospect of a different experience. Then hope, expressed as unwavering faith, can open an awareness of all possibilities. In the face of doubt about the likelihood of another's perception, providers may believe that any extraordinary measures are a delusion. Some practitioners may think it's an illusion, but spiritual beings and those who believing they cocreate their own reality disagree (Chapter 2). If beliefs shape reality and one person holds a different belief than another, then whose convictions are true? Many clinicians have seen people given a few months to live only to worsen as if heeding the expectations of a person in authority (nocebo). Healthcare workers can maintain an awareness of phraseology to avoid facing potential counterconditioning situations.

As life can hinge on risk versus benefits and omission versus commission, what are the mutual options? For many years, a physician applied for a clinical drug trial for his cancer patients but was denied. Under the 2015 Texas Right to Try law, he successfully treated some patients given 3-6 months to live. (Ebrahim Delpassand, 2016). In 2018, the United States Congress passed the Right to Try Act, allowing many terminally ill patients a chance to access investigational medical treatments. Doctor Delpassand was grateful for the ability to help patients through these therapies, which offered hope and quality of life to many of his patients. (Ebrahim Delpassand, 2021). This perspective held the space for life when a patient and provider never gave up.

Upon reflecting on my patient's journey to survivorship, this nurse stopped myopically perceiving personal beliefs supersedes another's. My logical mind may not have comprehended how or why unexplainable occurrences occur, but they do (Chapter 8). One person may dismiss miracles as unscientific, unproven, and unnatural, while another can view them as natural and certain. Therefore, since beliefs shape reality, both experiences can be perceived as authentic. Whether or not we believe something, it is real when it impacts someone's life. Pain sensations and other symptoms are felt whether a cause for them is found or not. There are new perspectives of idiopathic pain and other established chronic conditions (Chapter 6). My former patient never let a diagnosis, or anyone's opinion dictate her healing path; however, not all patients are as resilient.

This ICU experience had a profound impact on me, spurring many questions. "Had anyone else been open to understanding why this patient believed what they did?" "Did they wonder what happened after her extended hospital confinement?" "How did this patient perceive their state of health?" "Stable in managing chronic conditions, or were those eventually eclipsed by her personal beliefs?" "Could a person be deemed healthy while living with a medical condition?" The WHO Constitution redefined health to reflect "a state of complete physical, mental, and social well-being and not merely the absence of disease or infirmity." (WHO, 2017). Some may perceive this standard to mean that in order to be healthy, one must always live entirely within all these states. In my experience, most patients have expressed their state of being as either being ill or healthy.

Throughout time, various concepts and interpretations of health have existed. Medicine can consider establishing a unifying concept of the health objective, as medical lexicons, general dictionaries, and government organizations' versions vary. Otherwise, clinicians and patients can apply their own significance. Composite health definitions describe health as feeling well and devoid of illness. Is a person considered healthy if they are living with a diagnosed medical condition? The Merriam-Webster Dictionary describes health as being of "sound mind, body, and spirit." Can medicine acknowledge and address the deficiencies of a noncorporeal entity or soul within each being? Some ancient cultures have viewed "health as a balance between a person and the environment, the unity of soul and body, and the natural origin of disease." (Svalastog et al., 2017)

What does health mean to both the provider and the patient? Are their definitions the same for health, healing, and disease? A composite legal definition describes disease as a change in bodily functioning, characterized by specific symptoms or disabilities as diagnosed by a licensed provider. The medical community views chronic diseases as conditions that need to be managed rather than cured. This approach shifts the providers' focus from demanding the development of long-term solutions that address underlying disease (Chapter 6).

Is it possible for patients to meet the various definitions of health? Providers generally classify patients as being in either a favorable (healthy) or unfavorable (diseased) state, and disease as indicating bodily dysfunction or disability. Providers can perceive a malfunctioning body part as distinct from the rest of the functioning ones. This viewpoint prevents practitioners from perceiving the body as an interconnected whole. Patients and providers perceive wellness when functional capacity is restored, such as a fractured bone or when symptoms are resolved after a body organ is surgically removed. Is this accurate, or are practitioners overlooking the multidimensional causes of disease and the factors that contribute to healing (Chapter 6)?

There are disagreements within medicine about dysfunction arising from a disease state. Some practitioners believe there are bidirectional influences of psychosocial dimensions influencing disease. Therefore, addressing these underlying issues can lead to healing and health maintenance. However, these dimensions are not always recognized. How can providers and patients make informed decisions if they do not understand the origins of their conditions?

Currently, some people use different approaches to reach their perception of wellness. Personal values, nutritional and lifestyle education, and the mapping of one's care commitments may be seen as helping. However, since in-depth nutritional education is not sufficiently covered in medical and professional healthcare schools, a referral to a licensed clinician certified in lifestyle medicine may be considered. Many patients are seeking holistic care practices for disease prevention and healing. Some believe the healthcare systems (chapter 5) recognizing that unresolved trauma influences emotions, which affects the physical layer. Western Medicine has been inching toward viewing and treating each patient as a whole being. Currently, this practice defaults to doctors of osteopathy, naturopaths, and CAM practitioners operating within a whole-person approach. What study conclusions will emerge from the National Center for Complementary and Integrative Health (NCCIH), the NCCIH Strategic Plan 2021-2025 (Chapter 5)? Will transparent findings aid current practice and medical textbook authors in translating information for medical and ancillary health field texts and providing authoritative advice?

Some medical texts emphasize that socio-environmental elements influence health but don't fully address these and other broader human aspects. Some biomedical textbooks have been identified by researchers as being diluted due to undisclosed conflict-of-interest (COI) issues including payments from medical industry groups. While private and government research articles are accessible for the review of these issues, currently, there are not always permissions for reuse. Perceptions of these practices have left many prospective health professionals questioning the wholeness and reliability of their reference books. Due to the influence of perceived indisputable authoritative texts disclosure of COI seems compulsory. Will these concerns prompt respective professional associations to thoroughly review medical text transparency through an impartial research investigation? Investigating specified reference book issues and discrepancies enhances the ability to live the patient-provider healthcare intention.

Some health organizations and researchers believe that the interrelationship between biological factors, environmental influences, and, at times, spiritual elements contribute to both health and disease states. To avoid negative outcomes, it is necessary to provide training to assess for spiritual needs. (Harrad et al., 2019). In addition to the physical assessment, a more comprehensive psychosocial and spiritual assessment reflecting the reason for presenting complaints could be evaluated for standardization. Spiritual assessments are required in certain circumstances at Joint Commission-accredited facilities. (Joint Commission, 2022). If psychosocial and spiritual elements can catalyze illness (chapter 6), then these types of standard assessments appear to be merited.

What is the purpose of each professional interaction? Are the perspectives of the provider and patient congruent about the expected outputs of care? Providers don't offer a choice of symptom relief or appraisal of all disease constituents to reach the root causes of illness (Chapter 6). However, many patients and some healthcare professionals perceive medical practice as operating in this way. Many medical consumers are seeking ways to permanently correct pain and suffering without having to accept the perceived impossible. When pain-relieving remedies don't consistently target nociceptive responses and subjective neuropathic sensations, many are disappointed.

If providers focus on pain relief in one bodily area, an underlying factor elsewhere in the body can go undetected and unaddressed. Pain originating in one body part can radiate to (signal) another. The energy behind the symptom must be recognized to initiate precise treatment (Chapter 6). The persistence of chronic disease symptoms and disability has driven some of the global population to find other healing measures, whether medical industry-supported or not. Some people point to the lifestyle physicians (Preface) who have reversed some chronic diseases, disparate transparent research papers, and documentation of those who overcame terminal diagnoses by cure (spontaneous remission). Many providers join patients in their frustrations and have perceived beyond certain care standards (Preface).

Reflecting upon one former ICU patient changed my view of holistic therapies from skeptical to inquisitive. Perceptions expanded through open-mindedness and nonjudgment. The perceived fate of a human being holds significant power, especially when an individual or a group recognizes that another's projected limitations may become reality.

Education and experience lead clinicians to advise patients that chronic diseases are irreversible or incurable. Despite the researchers' findings of the root causes of many diseases and potential interventions, (all chapters), this belief remains dominant. Greater awareness, which fosters a higher vibrational energy, generates collective inspiration for a higher perspective (Preface). Will this shift in perspective encourage the medical community to explore these possibilities and move beyond traditional beliefs?

Practitioners often overlook the significant role perception plays in shaping their decisions. By acknowledging how both personal and collective perceptions can reshape reality, practitioners can start to challenge assumptions and expand their perspectives. This heightened awareness allows licensed practitioners to approach situations with enhanced clarity and make more informed decisions that reflect their authentic values and objectives. Ultimately, leveraging this awareness can transform challenges into opportunities, enriching both personal pursuits and professional endeavors.

Perspectives on the information thus far may vary, but as the coming chapters respond, each person chooses their beliefs and their truth.

# Chapter 2

## Perception: Reality Versus Illusions

"We don't see things as they are, we see them as we are.
~ Anais Nin

"All our knowledge has its origins in our perceptions."
~ Leonardo da Vinci

"So far as the mathematics refer to reality, they are not certain.
And so far as they are certain, they do not refer to reality."
~ Albert Einstein

"Reality is created by the mind; we can change our reality, by
changing our mind." ~ Plato

"It's not what you look at that matters it's what you see."
~ Henry David Thoreau

Everyone was spellbound while witnessing the impossible in New York City that evening. The audience continued acquiescing to the psychological techniques of the Magic Show's perception matrix by applauding deception. As the amplified sound of hand-shredded newspaper reverberated throughout the theater, everyone collectively accepted the unbelievable. Such sensory input, filtering through each being, compromised our veridical perceptions, constituting shared truth. In alignment with philosopher Maurice Merleau-Ponty, this demonstrated a "unification of visual, auditory, and sensory perceptions influencing belief." (Moya, 2014). Like children, we preferred to see real magic rather than illusions.

In real life, how can the extraordinary become a reality? Why do miraculous events seem to happen only to others? "Belief-reinforced awareness becomes our biochemistry." (Rao et al., 2009), thus reality. If this is the case, then through this mechanism, anyone can alter their circumstances. Nelson Mandela said: "It always seems impossible until it's done." Interestingly, many people hold false memories about this man and other historical events. The "Mandela Effect" emerged when many people recalled events differently from how they occurred or remembered events that never took place. Personal realities were created as some believed Mandela died in prison in the 1980s, not in 2013 as recorded. There are also misperceptions about Smokey the Bear, as the fire prevention campaign bear's name is Smokey Bear. The counterfactual (Palminteri, et al., 2017), may arise during encoding of the learning experience helping to promote illusions. Thus, the mere perception of events can influence belief and reality (chapter 5). Then perception can profoundly impact the scientific research sector and the judicial and medical systems, as people witnessing the same event can perceive and interpret it differently. So, how can anyone exert personal power (command of oneself, not over others) to dispel illusions?

Personal authority exists by living in the conscious perception of directing stimuli for subconscious processing. Not engaging in one's usual automatic reactions to people or situations including illness supports the natural capacity to access other experiences. People are subject to significant manipulation of perception in marketing, the many types of politics, and health matters. False or unsubstantiated claims presented as real can and have changed personal and public perceptions. The repetitiveness of assertions, whether actual or not, is and has been influential. Then, within the continued influence effect, misinformation survives even after correction.

Alteration strategies within the means of assistive devices enhancing perception are viewed as improving sensory processing and perceptual experiences. Though, can natural human encoding be improved? Some researchers have found that guided imagery and visualization can influence physiological processes. Positive outcomes were related to physical and psychological and perhaps this method can be useful "in the prevention and/or management of chronic disease." (Giacobbi et al., 2017).

The concept of healing encompasses the tenet of beliefs influencing perceptions. This paradigm influences every aspect of life, including conduct (chapter 4), healing, and wellness maintenance (chapter 8). As perception creates reality (Carbon, 2014), personal authority is exerted in whichever one is chosen. One block to well-being is the propensity to react to and align more with negative information. However, negativity bias may lead to irrational decisions (Molins et al., 2022). Then, dissociating from negativity bias (through mindfulness) may help in connecting to personal truth.

Past experiences can significantly impact decisions, potentially influenced by biases from previous choices (Bornstein et al., 2017). Perceptual impetus, involving both top-down attention (endogenous) and bottom-up attention (exogenous), is "mediated by at least partially distinct neural substrates." (Banerjee et al., 2019) (chapter 6). What accounts for the tendency of people to believe in optical illusions, chimeras, and magic acts despite their obvious falsity? Ulric Neisser's theory of the 'perceptual cycle' proposed a process for anticipating events. (Martínez-Pernía, 2020). His model was applied to understand the decision-making processes of mass transit operators. However, it is also relevant to the medical profession, as human perceptions and cognitive information can lead to critical errors from incorrect decisions (chapter 5).

Everything is processed and validated through personal perception that constitutes belief. However, beliefs are not always facts; they are simply things a person chooses to accept as truth. Thus, living by what is synthesized as fact based on past experiences, current mental, emotional, and physiological states, and collective and personal beliefs help shape thoughts. One's thoughts, perceptions, and emotional state reside in the subconscious mind, emerging from associations that reinforce personal truth (one's personal knowledge of reality). Authority figures confirming perpetuating an action can produce a sense of normalization even if those initiatives don't create a desired result. This phenomenon can lead individuals or organizations to continue pursuing ineffective strategies simply because they have become accustomed to them. Viewing the same reality as absolute truth obstructs the need for any modification, establishing it as a constant. Such an attitude stifles the opportunity for realizing innovation and improvement. In the past, people were skeptical of the realities of inventors, visionaries, and artists. Now, their visions can be perceived as having been grounded in chimera.

"Perception selects and makes the world you see. It literally picks it out as the mind directs. The laws of size and shape and brightness would hold, perhaps, if other things were equal. They are not equal. For what you look for you are far more likely to discover than what you would prefer to overlook." (ACIM, T-21V.1-5, p. 456). Some have conformed to the perceptual reality of others by succumbing to their limiting statements (nocebo effect) (Hansen & Zech, 2019). The power of perception can often shape one's experience in profound ways, where negative expectations can lead to a belief as truth, promoting fear and adverse outcomes. Whatever one thinks, disbelieves, continually repeats, or believes about oneself and others often translates to personal reality.

As a charge nurse in a psychiatric hospital, one patient's philosophical beliefs dictated their care. My patient (a retired psychiatrist) refused a physical examination until they understood the point of view of the on-call doctor. The assessment commenced when the young physician asserted the deductive reasoning approach would guide his clinical judgment. The patient suggested that using an inductive reasoning approach would have prevented the exam, thereby delaying their emergency room transfer. As this facility diagnosed patients' personal realities, standard manuals guiding the diagnosis and correction of a mental condition (an altered state of consciousness) did not always account for one's truth at the point of personal perception. "What perception sees and hears appears to be real because it permits into awareness only what conforms to the wishes of the perceiver." (ACIM, Preface, p. x). The recognition of comprehensive multifactorial influences affecting all aspects of physical and mental health was not standardized. To fit in with the perception of society, patients meeting the existing criteria for mental disorders agreed to specialized treatments like psychotherapy, medication, and sometimes electroconvulsive therapy. Despite chosen therapies, some maintained certainty that their perceptions of reality were accurate. However, the judges of correct reality differed, as they did not personally experience the emprises of others.

Not everyone having phantasms supports a diagnosis of a mental disorder. Trauma, stress, prescribed or non-prescribed substances, and some believe a connection with a deity, can account for altered perceptions. Decades ago, coding for a religious or spiritual problem did not exist. Since then, one diagnostic code for it suggested a "differential diagnosis between spiritual and psychopathological pathology." (Lindahl et al., 2020). This was then replaced with another code for religious or spiritual counseling. Spiritual distress does not include the millions of people worldwide who believe that the Holy Spirit resides within them, that they are an aspect of God, or those who hold personal religious or spiritual beliefs. Some mental health or medical practitioners may not believe in another's self-directed cognitive behavior. This awareness highlights the significance of nonjudgement to prevent countertransference. A spiritual assessment is required for those receiving professional services for specific diagnoses at Joint Commission-accredited hospitals. (Joint Commission, 2022). Many people around the world use religious or spiritual practices to find peace and healing. Thus, a spiritual assessment can be considered at every health-related visit to learn more about each person's preferences.

Some find it challenging to relate to anyone experiencing anything unidentifiable, intangible, or beyond the human senses as being real. As truth is experienced differently, can anyone's spiritual or religious identity be judged? Though, some people continue choosing to discredit another's perception of the supernatural. Vivid dreams, chimeras, miracles, and placebo study participants experiencing real effects after ingesting a pill without any active ingredient exemplify people experiencing reality differently. If reality is subjective, can there be a universal description of it? Or can the definitions provided by organizations, philosophers, and dictionaries establish a general sense of certainty? "Reality is changeless." (ACIM, T-30.VIII.1:2, p. 643). "Reality is that which never changes, which is absolute, unlimited, and is never contradicted by any other thing or experience." (Swami Krishnananda).

Some people have reported experiencing the reality of synesthesia as they taste color or smell music and sounds. While medicine does not classify these sensory crossovers as psychogenic or as a mental illness, idiopathic pain sensations and symptoms are sometimes classified as such. Virtual or complex changes in sensory input can alter one's perception of reality. Years after a surgical below-the-knee amputation, my patient complained of pain in his lower leg "Phantom limb pain is considered a neuropathic pain, and most treatment recommendations are based on recommendations for neuropathic pain syndromes." (Subedi & Grossberg, 2011). Though, whether an amputation was due to an accident or a surgical procedure resulting in a missing body part, it can be perceived as trauma and potentially classified as posttraumatic stress disorder (PTSD). Some licensed mental health professionals offer cognitive or other PTSD therapies.

"Perception is a choice and not a fact. But on this choice depends far more than you may realize as yet. For on the voice you choose to hear, and on the sights you choose to see, depends entirely your whole belief in what you are.* "Perception is a witness to this but to this, and never to reality. Yet it can show you the conditions in which awareness of reality is possible, or those where it could never be." (ACIM, T-21V.1, p. 456). "Reality needs no cooperation from you to be itself. But your awareness of it needs your help because it is your choice. Listen to what the ego says, and see what it directs you see, and it is sure that you will see yourself as tiny, vulnerable, and afraid. You will experience depression, a sense of worthlessness, and feelings of impermanence and unreality. You will believe that you are helpless prey to forces far beyond your own control, and far more powerful than you. And you will think the world you made directs your destiny. For this will be your faith. But never believe because it is your faith it makes reality." (ACIM, T-21V.2, p. 456). The choice of perspective, including one's belief of who they are (chapter 8) is powerful.

Beliefs significantly influence perceptions, potentially leading to experiencing illusions as reality. This is evident in the story of a person who thought they were dead. As the patient and their provider agreed that the dead don't bleed, they settled on a method of proof. During the successful blood draw, the patient reinforced their belief by declaring that dead people bleed. While this is a fictional account, the walking corpse syndrome is a real and documented phenomenon. In 2016, an accident survivor with severe injuries was interviewed on Good Morning Britain (Good Morning Britain, 2016). As this man believed he was not alive, his healthcare provider diagnosed him with Cotard's syndrome. He recovered after meeting and engaging with someone else with the same diagnosis. This can be understood through phenomenology, which involves viewing situations from the perspective of someone who has had similar experiences. This concept is a core principle in many support groups.

Phenomenology is, "The science of the essence of consciousness." ~ Edmund Husserl.

At some point, everyone has experienced an alteration in visual perception. Edgar Rubin's Mind Influences Matter depicts two faces versus a vase on contrasting backgrounds. As in life, the illustration's depiction of only one object at a time depends on the location of the focus. In a functional magnetic resonance imaging experiment, researchers measured participants' stimulus, processing, and interpretation of information (Ishizu & Zeki, 2014). Subjects pressed a button upon experiencing the reversal of a figure. Perceiving these reversals activated the brain areas believed to be involved in brief perceptual conflict resolution. In another experiment involving brain mapping with magnetoencephalography, the researcher concluded that prior expectations of stimuli can alter perception (Ishizu, 2013).

Top-down modulation can produce anticipation of specific upcoming catalysts. "We do not see the external world as it really is; rather, we see it as we think it should be depending on available information." (Ishizu, 2013). Another alteration in visual brain processes influencing perception is due to the Moon Illusion where the Moon appears larger when viewed near the horizon (NASA). Once, a teacher sent the class out into the hallway. Upon returning, we experienced an illusion when we saw "Paris in the Sprigtime" written on the chalkboard. We unanimously recited "Paris in the Springtime." Perhaps the Gestalt Law of Closure allowed everyone to see the word as complete.

Sometimes, people project onto others what is within themselves. Choosing to see things from a broader perspective by avoiding preconceptions, biases, judgments, and self-projection prevent perceptual errors. Self-projection occurs when a personal belief transferred to another creates a false reality (an unwanted illusion). The chain reaction continues as one relinquishes personal authority, cultivating a hopeless perception. One's authenticity overtaking another's facilitates a false sense of reality. Authority figures are influential when they project their beliefs onto others. Insertion of professional and personal perceptions (opinions), or judgments can foster illusions that potentially shape undesired outcomes (nocebo) (Hansen & Zech, 2019). Then one can potentially influence another's reality to match theirs (Introduction). When one directs their energy in judgment or opinions, objective assessment and assistance are blurred.

Criticism generates negative emotions and changes vibrations (chapter 8), fueling anger, hate, and hostility, allowing chemical messengers to create new conditions or exacerbate existing ones (chapter 6). Judgments can separate people from one another, allowing discord and the dissolution of relationships. The tendency to make value judgments can alter the dynamics in any romantic, personal, or professional relationship. The habit of judging denies another's freedom of personal expression (appearance, choices, etc.), yielding unnecessary suffering. When others make assumptions about someone or a situation, choosing to rise above them helps with objectivity. A broader perspective allows us to see the nuances of each situation rather than hastily forming opinions.

Stereotyping, a form of judgment that divides and inflicts harm while diminishing individuals, stands in opposition to the essence of shared humanity. As individuals are categorized based on their state, country, political party, or religion they are confined to the beliefs imposed by the judger. Instead of allowing each person to express their authenticity, selective perceptions that form assumptions terminate the conversation, obstructing a potential understanding of the truth. Sincere questions assist in clarifying the beliefs of individuals across cultures, regions, nonpartisan views, and spiritual beliefs (such as some Jewish people who believe in Jesus). Throughout recorded history, fear has been the driving force behind the control of others, persuading them to harbor animosity toward individuals or stereotypical groups. This dominion intends to alienate people from one another, their spiritual source, personal truth, and sovereignty. One might wonder how this perception is beneficial to them.

Anyone controlling (action) others loses their freedom to the opposite result (reaction). When evaluating another, one may see a reflection of themselves and retaliate. One's anger and hate can encourage others to believe falsehoods about another person or a group of people (gossip). Making others look bad seemingly elevates oneself or a group above others, inclining superiority and exclusion. Historical perspectives illustrate how such beliefs have cultivated unified malice, leading to human destruction. As individuals surrender their identities and freedom, they feel separate from others and start opposing them. This prevailing atmosphere stifles personal expression and complicates the pursuit of individual truth.

So, how can one break free from subjugation and conditioned beliefs and discover their truth? Establishing truth requires introspection, reflection on experiences, and an openness to the truth, whatever it is. Genuine truth does not fear questioning but withstands scrutiny, is not influenced by opinion, and retains its validity. This differs from an agenda-driven truth that involves elements of control, force, hostility, and bias. When truth is not distorted or manipulated by another's agenda, it is easier to establish trust. This insight can enable people to reconnect with their authentic selves and acknowledge their shared humanity (chapter 10).

Open-mindedness, nonjudgment, and a heightened perspective (Preface) reduces bias. In alignment with philosophers Locke and Hume, a teacher once advised, "Don't believe anything you hear and only half of what you see." This guidance motivated me to seek the truth for myself and understand the reasons behind others' beliefs and actions. Did a person or group express something or act out of fear? And to learn what perceptions might be shaping another's reality. If reality is experienced differently, can a standard certainty truly exist? "Nothing real can be threatened" "Nothing unreal exists." (ACIM, Preface, p. x). The real and true never change only one's beliefs about them do, creating the space for establishing truth or defending illusions.

Synthesizing and internalizing experiences solidifies our perception of reality through human senses. The act of hearing and interpreting words carries significant power. When negative beliefs are imposed on children, those who are mentally, emotionally, or physically ill, and the elderly, it can distort their understanding of reality and truth. Such individuals may feel compelled to conform to a distorted reality when pressured by those in authority. This was evident in childhood, as my parents often reacted to many situations with judgment, anger, and yelling. Consequently, internalizing their words and actions, led to feelings of fear and shame. Eventually, personal empowerment emerged by recognizing and embracing my truth, rather than theirs (below).

"Misperceptions produce fear and true perceptions foster love, but neither brings certainty because all perception varies."

(ACIM, T-3.111.8 p. 40). It can be easy to conform to another's reality if one believes their repetitious belittling statements. Those viewed in authority as holding ultimate power at the time can continue to have influence even decades later. Then one may try to make sense of and survive childhood experiences permeating their consciousness. It can be challenging to pivot from the core beliefs of authority figures and adverse childhood experiences (ACEs, chapter 6). For me, internalizing what another held as true did not have to remain a personal reality. My perceptions were changed by choosing different thoughts, beliefs, and by not reliving negative experiences. "Our beliefs provide the script to write or rewrite the code of our reality." (Rao et al., 2009).

The methods described below are reflective of my personal healing experience. Consult your personal licensed mental healthcare provider when seeking to reconcile past traumatic events. The mere presence of me and my sisters triggered Dad, who transformed his energy into anger and violence. Therefore, he was never in his power, although he thought he was. Without excusing his actions, perhaps he was reliving the acts of his tormentor(s). In early adulthood, the cadre of mental health professionals could not obliterate my past. One therapist's analogy of carrying my childhood experiences around like an anchor was correct. Each time the traumatic experiences were recounted, the past and present became interchangeable. These mental images helped me to recreate and relive traumatic memories, invoking the same past chemicals in my then-current physical body.

It can be challenging to break free from conditioned beliefs, especially when they go unrecognized and are reinforced through physical abuse. For me, he first became triggered when I attempted to contribute to a conversation, interpreting this action as talking back. He then justified his actions whenever he sensed I was about to speak. Each time rage coursed through his body, he experienced an intense surge of energy that compelled him to act on impulse. With each occurrence, Mom retreated.

These encounters helped me retreat into a quiet world and without a way to relay real concerns to my parents. I wondered, "Why were we being controlled by fear and humiliation?" My sister Barbara, who had her run-ins with Dad, recounted what Mom had told her. After Dad's father died, his mother felt unable to support two children and asked another family to care for her three-year-old son. During that time, he had experienced abuse. Perhaps he felt the density of guilt and shame for whatever may have altered his childhood innocence.

A disconnect of a sense of self perpetuated a cycle of family dysfunction and shared suffering. Channeling anger through his being continued to trigger a primal fight-or-flight response, signaling his cells to fight each other. Among the many maladies he suffered were a heart attack, arrhythmia, and dementia, forgetting all abuses he suffered and caused. Later in life, I observed other people exhibiting unresolved emotional conflicts eventually contending with chronic medical conditions. I pondered whether consistent negative emotional experiences influencing sympathetic responses led to chronic disease. This and other questions prompted a decade-long research inquiry into the potential connection between emotional well-being and physical health.

When Dad passed, our mom said, "All his demons went with him." In a dream, he told me, "Well, I made it, but they aren't making it easy for me." At the time, this was perceived as a fitting response. Choosing to see things from a different perspective helped me see the illusion of taking Dad's words and actions personally. His expressions of anger did not arise because of me or my siblings. Devoid of self-love from traumatic childhood experiences (chapter 6), he likely saw himself, his family, and God as separate. Since he could not experience happiness and peace, we were being denied them. Being separate from his truth created constant personal and family discord. Dad likely demeaned our value because he felt worthless. He unfortunately chose to control us through fear (false evidence appearing real), intimidation, and force.

I stopped my reactions to perceived immutable past events by changing the energy associated with them. Another Reiki practitioner guided me to a practice of serenity where I imagined my deceased parents hearing me talking to them. In this realm, they had no power. After thanking them for providing for me, I expressed my truth. In an act of self-love, I forgave all illusions because their actions were unrelated to me and did not define me. This mental exercise helped a false reality disappear. Perceiving myself not as a victim but as a worthy being, changed the perception of my past. Previously, I had coped by visualizing a hired bodybuilder standing behind me during mealtimes (when Dad's anger would trigger). In that reality, the mere presence of my imaginary buff bodyguard prevented any calamity.

From the perspective of compassion, a positive outcome resulted after the fact. I came to understand my personal power. This feeling lifted an emotional burden, allowing me to live free from a different perspective, which was one facet in restoring my emotional and physical wellness. However, some professional mental health organizations and providers don't agree with creating false memories. Though, some neuroscientific papers indicate that the counterfactual can be helpful as scientists learn more about how the brain and consciousness are connected. Neuroscience may assist with guided mental imagery for emotional processing that influences both mental and physical health (Van Hoeck et al., 2015) and may prevent unwanted memories from resurfacing (Clark & Mackay, 2015). This area of study may be beneficial in addressing trauma and addiction, as research concentrates on learned experiences (encoding) that involve memory substrates stored within a neural ensemble (engram) (Ramsey et al., 2023). It may also prove useful in fear conditioning models. (Iqbal et al., 2023). Can changing memories (beliefs) impact the chemical and physical properties associated with engrams, thereby altering an encoded experience to help cure chronic diseases (chapter 6)?

The past holds no authority; there is only power in one's present perspectives and choices. Affirmations (Finley et al., 2018) and a different perspective possibly deactivated my negative feedback loop by altering my brain's responses. These affirmations reinforced the truth of my deservingness of healing. One such declaration was, "I release all anger and hostility from my body, heart, mind, and spirit and accept only peace." Consult your qualified licensed healthcare provider(s) about their views on guided or self-guided imagery, visualization, and other psychological techniques. It helped me to see my dad from a different perspective while understanding that his truth was not mine.

However, one can consider removing themselves from an abusive or dangerous situation and seeking professional assistance by contacting local authorities, personal licensed healthcare providers, emergency services, and, in the United States (U.S.), the National Domestic Violence Hotline for support. Outside of the U.S., check your country's government and domestic violence websites for the appropriate contact information. While not condoning Dad's abusive actions, he likely could not have realized the full current and future impact of his choices. Some oppressors acquit themselves with the "I was abused" defense, though Dad always had the simple power to choose his beliefs and conduct. Years later, I was in a situation where there was no escape. This experience helped me to see beyond that circumstance and find my power.

While flying in a small private plane, I asked my pilot friend why he sabotaged the flight. His response was, "I want to see if I can recover it from a stall." My sympathetic nervous system automatically deployed. I had to make a quick decision. Either act on my true feelings of fear, terror, and anger by freaking out and sounding off or not. In this fight-or-flight situation, the fight became whether or not to display the above true emotions. Immediately, I chose to project a false calm exterior, while trying to suppress the opposing internal set of automatic signals and responses. At that moment, life hinged on not distracting the pilot; thus, matching his calm demeanor would allow him to focus on reversing his actions. Mind-body techniques in silent prayer helped me stay in my power during this terrifying experience. Bottom-up and top-down processes maintained emotional regulation. My heart was no longer going to beat out of my chest. By shifting my consciousness, the emotions experienced were regulated by self-directed neuroplasticity. The plane responded to the pilot's matter-of-fact attention with a safe landing. I did not seek retribution.

Attempting to get even with or get back at someone can create a barrier to healing. This collapses power, creating a false sense of control. Judging others and not allowing them to explain their side often leads to misperceptions. This scenario brings to mind personal stories of parents rejecting their children and vice versa. Parents and kids have reciprocally condemned the choices of partners (judging personal expression) and other personal decisions, including divorce, leading to disowning them (control by withholding access and love). Falsehoods, misunderstandings, and opinions have led to estrangement within families, perpetuating anger. Though, there are serious considerations of having someone back in one's life, especially if it is perceived as unloving and unsafe. Everyone holds an unconscious connection and association and significance upon hearing certain words.

Cymatics musician Nigel Stanford demonstrates the connection between sound waves and the physical world. (Stanford, 2021). In communication, words, tone, and vibration enhance the interpretation and perception of their meaning. Nonverbal communication is also powerful. One provider's facial expression conveyed judgment of my usage of a complementary therapy. These therapies may be seen as unfounded, and medicine should only be offering that which is scientifically proven. Is every intervention delivered consistently safe, effective, and devoid of short-term or long-term effects? Can we solely attribute healing to certain standard treatment sets, or are there other factors at play? A real-time quantum healing video has documented the healing of a bladder tumor (Braden, 2011). Is it possible for a person's beliefs to hold such power, where is the scientific evidence to back this up, and will researchers commit to potentially replicating this scenario?

It may feel unnatural to question everything we have always considered true. However, challenging long-held beliefs can lead to reassessing assumptions, resulting in a more informed perspective. Selective filtering of information shapes personal beliefs, thoughts, decisions, and actions. By acknowledging the power of perception, we become aware of its ability to distort or enhance our understanding of reality. This awareness allows one to look beyond preconceived notions and discover new perspectives. Understanding personal reality begins with recognizing that our perceptions are not always objective truths but rather reflections of subjective experiences.

Insights from the next chapter highlight the importance of research effectiveness in creating evidence-based guidelines and best practices underpinning medical practice. Recognizing the necessity for accurate scientific conclusions reinforces the integrity of professional judgment, ensuring that practitioners can navigate complex clinical scenarios with confidence. This commitment to precise research practices enhances the credibility of the medical product and fortifies trust between healthcare providers and patients. Ultimately, the synthesis of these elements underscores a shared responsibility in advancing healthcare quality and safeguarding public health.

# Chapter 3

## The Scope and Efficacy of Scientific Research

**"Research is seeing what everybody else has seen and thinking what nobody else has thought."** ~ Albert Szent-Györgyi

**"To maximize the benefit to society, you need to not just do research but do it well."** ~ Doug Altman

**"A new scientific truth does not triumph by convincing its opponents and making them see the light, but rather because its opponents eventually die, and a new generation grows up that is familiar with it."** ~ Max Planck

**"Science is nothing but perception."** Plato

**"Once you know, you are responsible."** ~ Austin Frakt

Harm has been an unfortunate consequence of conflicting study conclusions in biomedical literature. Since its inception, scientific investigations founding medical advances have faced significant challenges. How can scientists overcome recurring research objections and avoid common pitfalls to uphold scientific integrity? Or is the process of establishing evidence for therapeutics already considered exceptional? While there are apparent successes across the healthcare spectrum, many biomedical investigators are pursuing the correction of well-known issues in scientific investigation to strengthen its foundation and, thus, its output. To be committed, they can see it as their duty to stay objective so that they can devise empirical interpretations that help them make decisions that support the medical profession's intention, mission, and vision. This fulfills the promise of furthering critical thinking, truth in science, and knowledge of disease pathogenesis and justifiable interventions.

This chapter highlights the burdens of biomedical researchers within the investigative process in meeting the above goals. Their views enable a broader perspective on bridging gaps within biomedical scientific studies affecting evidence-based medicine (EBM) for clinical application and personal utilization. Their work implies humanitarian service in helping to identify root causes of diseases that lead to quality interventions. Since no specific authority evaluates and determines the veracity of all scientific claims, it becomes the charge of each clinician. Challenges arise for these final interpreters of research data that impact medical consumers. By developing a critical understanding of the methodologies employed in studies, practitioners can better discern the validity of findings and effectively apply them in their practice. The interface of biomedical research papers and practice can appear consistent even with the presentation of previous and new divergent findings. Is this representative of provider time constraints, exegesis of conclusions, or resistance to change?

How interested are research article reviewers in the intrinsic motivation. (Di Domenico & Ryan, 2017) and personal beliefs of each investigator? What is the perception of the practitioner while reading a research paper? Is there a holistic view of the research enterprise, appraising disparate results to avoid one-size-fits-all recommendations? Does selective perception bias lead to fixed responses? Consequently, the inconsistencies in professional interpretations of biomedical papers may result in varying concepts of implementation. This makes understanding the complex processes that result in bringing knowledge into collective existence essential. Information within this chapter is gathered from government agencies, medical organizations, and many biomedical research papers, many in declaration of no conflict of interest (COI) or external funding. Health resources that are free from bias, rather than those with a hidden agenda, influence guideline recommendations. They also support a scientific foundation for clinical actions and promote well-informed shared decision-making.

Any form of bias can influence a researcher's conclusions and recommendations. When examining COI statements, readers can discern whether stakeholder benefits may have influenced critical outcomes. Biases undermine bioethical principles in respect to "autonomy, beneficence, nonmaleficence, and justice." (Mousavi, 2024). Partisanship is not immune to individual papers, systematic reviews, and meta-analyses. Publication bias can distort validity of research. (Olsson TM, Sundell, 2023). Publishing only positive data can compromise other researchers' experiments, and harm may result from distorted conclusions. Not publishing negative study results can diminish the full scope of risk of harms versus benefits. Is the practice of omitting negative conclusions contributing to lag-time* science? Is publication bias accounting for the failure to replicate studies?

Furthermore, as a reviewer of a research study, limitations and other biases inherent in all studies may not be apparent. (Ross, 2019). Authors have identified limitations in the gold standard of randomized controlled trial (RCT) analysis. Many current medical practices are ineffective due to issues with RCT. (Herrera-Perez et al., 2019). Results by proxy may not consistently find the most common adverse effects of a treatment or consider people who have the same comorbidities. Additionally, healthy Phase 1 clinical trial participants' interpretations of correct reporting of bodily changes as harms have been questioned. (McManus et al., 2019). After a review of over 3000 RCTs published in three leading medical journals, 396 medical reversals were identified. (Herrera-Perez et al., 2019). The reevaluation resulted in changes to the guidelines for aspirin (NIH, 2019), hormone replacement therapy, and other standard recommendations.

Conflicting studies, which either warn of the cancer-causing effects of coffee or confirm its benefits, provide an emblematic example. Initially, concern was placed on the chemical components in coffee as potentially being carcinogenic. However, the likely causes of mucosal injury and esophageal cancer have changed. It is noted that hot beverage consumption (tea) ($\geq 65°C$) showed a significant risk of esophageal squamous cell carcinoma. (Luo & Ge, 2022).

According to numerous physicists, evidence in the scientific realm is provisional. According to Plato, "Science is nothing but perception." However, clinicians and the public can construe findings to imply complete infallibility and indisputable evidence in published papers. Clinicians have to overcome a plethora of issues when attempting to validate a study. A gold standard (even with RCT) cannot be established as, "It is impossible to know with 100% certainty what the truth is in any research question." (Ioannidis, 2005). Researchers then sit with the insoluble while attempting to establish knowledge within the scope of this mechanism.

Can the scientific method resolve conflicting beliefs between scientists and groups? Most ancient people accepted that the world was flat. Many now believe it is round or ellipsoid. (NORR, 2023). However, some individuals and groups continue to hold onto the original belief. Will consensus be reached, or can each view be reinforced by Einstein's general relativity theory or theory of gravity?

As general facts change, so does medical knowledge. Just as with chemical elements and drugs, there is a decay or half-life of knowledge over time. Dr. Burwell advised his medical students, "Half of what we are going to teach you is wrong, and half of it is right. Our problem is that we don't know which half is which." (Charles Sidney Burwell). Samuel Arbesman suggests that it takes 45 years to refute and overturn knowledge. (Arbesman, 2012). Scientometrics examines the connections between medical literature and scientific fields. (Jozi & Nourmohammadi, 2022). So, how has the medical community responded if it takes 45 years (the half-life of truth) to overturn just half of the medical knowledge (current standard reality)? How will they respond in the future? As general and biomedical facts constantly change, are medical systems keeping pace with them? Is the current foundation of medicine sustainable for establishing scientific authority in the future? This chapter further explores the features, idiosyncrasies, and potentials of this method, which currently serves as a means of acquiring evidence. Observing an impeccable scientific research process can prevent researchers from building upon previous potentially flawed conclusions.

Scientific Evaluation and Review of Claims in Health Care (SEaRCH™), uses several methods to evaluate product claims or interventions that work in healthcare. (Jonas et al., 2017). Some government groups and agencies use other expert panels to connect evidence with clinical guidance. (Jonas et al., 2017). These panels have their own strengths and weaknesses. "For the development of trustworthy guidelines there should be concordance between the quality (certainty) of the evidence and the strength of the recommendations." (Chong et al., 2023).

Scientific research conclusions and interpretations may satiate our curiosity or invite more questions when reviewing research author-cited study limitations or noting their absence. For unstable healthcare environments, it is crucial that the process establishing standards for health, prevention, and life-or-death decisions consider a diverse range of unbiased information. However, can we be certain that recent standards are genuinely based on the most current information? There is a considerable lag time* between scientific bench discoveries and integration into medical practice. Thus, there is a consistent delay in the dissemination and utilization of potentially the most current clinically effective problem-solving and therapeutic approaches. This limits diagnosticians in clinical question formation and appraising the most current information. Time lags* occur as research evidence endures years of safety reviews or numerous citations of an investigator's work. (Morris et al., 2011). Then can be a delay of 17 years before data from human subject clinical trials and translation into clinical practice. (Morris et al., 2011). How can the investigative paradigm improve as investigators empirically research methods for interventions deemed safe, efficacious, and cost-effective while contending with the "half-life of truth?" By recognizing that science is a dynamic process rather than a static collection of facts, researchers can consider the ultimate end of research.

What is the purpose of biomedical research? Is it to engage scientists in working to flawlessly create disease-specific antidotes? Can medical researchers and medical professionals consider the end goals of research as the ability to treat the underlying biomedical mechanisms of disease? Healing implies agreement that research has always sought the truth, whatever it is. Truth in science holds significant power in identifying the underlying mechanisms of disease and determining appropriate interventions. When clinicians and medical consumers don't realize desired healing, they may give up or search elsewhere. Effective communication about biomedical research commands consistency between the medical community and the public. Inconsistency between providers, the Internet, and other media outlets has vast implications for health guidance. Impeccable science practice is a powerful exploratory tool in establishing truth for safe and reliable clinical guidance. Understanding how conflicts emerge within it begins with examining the underpinnings of the investigative process. An exceptional process that contributes to the accuracy of interpreted results is required for precise knowledge.

Biomedical research investigators select a conceptual framework prior to data collection to support the design of the study type. Readers of scientific papers may take for granted that the best hypothesis question was asked and that different questions (curiosity without preconceived expectations) permitted drawing pure answers. Reviewing caveats regarding the strengths and limitations of the research design may help determine study validity.

Some researchers hold contrary views about the current null hypothesis statistical testing (NHST) model and cite its pitfalls. "More can be learned from data by evaluating specific expectations, or so-called *informative* hypotheses, than by testing the traditional null hypothesis." (Van de Shoot et al., 2011). That is, investigators can reject it when true (Type I error) or accept it when false (Type II error). (Banerjee et al., 2009). One can select statistical tests for validation in advance to help prevent errors. Generally, NHST variables have no effect (if they do, it may be by chance), while the alternate hypothesis assumes an effect. In evaluating a study, was the hypothesis question in the introduction answered in the conclusion? Do findings show correlations? Two correlated variables can show association but not necessarily cause-and-effect. (Kumar & Chong, 2018). Have researchers repeated and replicated experiments with similar subjects? Or can objective scientists refuting previous research, pose a new hypothesis question to bring them closer to different solutions?

Operating within a special interest framework may cause one to lose focus on the quality of medical investigation. When obtaining the same results, is it due to competitive issues (bias, funding, or other COIs)? "Misinterpretation of $P$-values and statistically significant test results persists also among persons who have substantial statistical education and who work professionally with statistics." (Lytsy et.al., 2022). Are these factors accounting for disparities in interpretations? How can we reconcile discrepancies when previous health recommendations touting benefits are then deemed ineffective or harmful? Are insurance payers covering gold standards based on potential process impairments, and investigators' beliefs or biases? While research intends to advance medical knowledge, significant process considerations exist.

One important consideration is understanding the quality of measurement tools used for data collection and analysis. Biostatisticians may be used for quality data oversight methods. Graphs, charts, and tables use statistical findings to represent the conclusions of corresponding values. "The type of statistical analysis performed" may account for study limitations. (Ross et al., 2019). Many authors and organizations emphasize the importance of reducing the probability (p-value) index to reduce issues of data analysis and interpretation. The P value is used in data analysis, however, there has been some misuse and misrepresentation of it. Especially in the presence of a poorly design. (Wang & Long, 2022). Do these factors thoroughly explain why same-subject studies have corroborating or differing results?

When reading a biomedical paper, one trusts in the objective performance of the study process from hypothesis to publication. And that the hypotheses were not changed after the interpretation of the results. The Open Science Collaboration (OSC) replicated 100 published psychology studies. They found that 97% of the original studies reported $p < .05$; only 36% of the replicated ones showed statistically significant results. The Open Science Framework (OSF) supports investigators in every aspect of the study process to enhance openness, integrity, and reproducibility. The Hawthorne Effect may affect the observational p-value result as behaviors can change from being observed. (Wu et al., 2018).

In 2015, Transparency and Openness Promotion (TOP) introduced eight modular standards for open and transparent research. Their standards in manuscript submission encourage pre-registration and registration of works and data sharing to improve communication and replication and reduce bias. The Top Factor metric reports the steps journals can take in implementing open science practices. The OSF describes its 24-page Journal Policies and Practices (TOP Guidelines) and asserts various categories expand to provide three levels of transparency.

According to the Open Science Framework authors (Mayo-Wilson et al. (2021), suggest that journals check to see if any open practices and TOP standards have been used and list the journals that agree to these standards. This can assist readers in assessing the study standards used. The Center for Open Science promotes the use of badges as incentives for open practices in medical journals. These certifications communicate knowledge within the research facility by publicly sharing methodology for better reproducibility. Transparency helps clarify the goals of medicine and the caregiver's role and serves as a clinical indicator and constant for evaluation.

Can any research organization account for perceptions in stereotyping, judgments, and assumptions that can lead to unconscious bias (UB)? These biases allow an unconscious researcher to generate conscious results. (Gopal et al., 2018). Can recognizing bias help other researchers to assess, recognize, and remediate another's UB? Will scientists follow this recommendation? While some use a test to detect implicit bias, some question if it is an "accurate measure of bias or a prediction of it." (Sukhera et al., 2019).

Research entities and guideline developers that adhere to their own conflict of interest policies and abstain from accepting industry funding help to eliminate perceptions of impropriety. Issues of COI prompted the Open Payments disclosure program to enhance research transparency and accountability. (openpaymentsdata.cms.gov). When reviewing a biomedical research article is potential partiality disclosed or derived from the COI statements? These biases may account for conflicting conclusions leading to contrary determination statements in same-subject papers.

As previously mentioned, clinicians consider RCT to be the most reliable source of evidence. Researchers prefer this method as it offers a clear understanding of how to establish the effectiveness of interventions. However, there are shortcomings of this design. Subjects with great differences (sampling bias) are not ideal populations, and ethically, humans cannot participate in harmful behaviors. Thus, many research authors agree that not all RCT conclusions can equate findings with indisputable evidence.

Additionally, research authors concur that the results of RCTs in lab settings may not necessarily translate to practice settings. If the RCT population differs from the real-world population, these trials won't be replicated. (Averitt et al., 2020).

Organizations can consider developing frameworks for generating applicable hypotheses for heterogenous trial populations. There are challenges and usefulness in using the mixed-methods research approach. (Regnault et al., 2017).

While some complex RCT evaluations incorporate qualitative research, these findings can be analyzed separately. Advocates of the mixed methods approach view them as helping to determine outcome variations.

Clinicians and patients only want to experience the benefits of published clinical trial results. It is essential to highlight the impact of established research biases. These elements compromise the quality of results and interpretations, profoundly affecting human outcomes. Many factors can account for discordance in analysis and interpretation. When evaluating studies, did the repeated study avoid selection bias by considering the exact make-up of study participants for that targeted population? A flawed design and defective instruments can change actual values, potentially leading to significant real-life consequences. All agencies involved in research must address all known issues to improve accuracy and transparency for the reliability of conclusions.

Practice guidelines from clinical trials can benefit from input from various medical professional disciplines. These clinicians may advance their practice through pragmatic trial approaches. Pragmatic trial designs using Pragmatic Explanatory Continuum Indicator Summaries (PRECIS) were developed to bridge perfect lab conditions and practice settings. (WWW.precis-2.org). The 5-point Oxford Quality Rating Scale in Cochrane reviews also depends on double-blind trials. Though this trial design benefits drug trials, it does not benefit all other study types. The Consolidated Standards of Reporting Trials (CONSORT) promotes recommendations in reporting randomized trials affecting healthcare decision-making (consort statement). Their 25-item checklist focuses on trial design, analysis, and interpretation.

Observational studies (cohort, case-control, or cross-sectional studies) may be considered in lieu of RCT. These studies can show correlations but do not necessarily establish cause and effect however, blinding may reduce observation bias in these studies. A tool for enhancing the presentation of observational study journal reporting is a collaborative 22-item checklist or Strengthening the Reporting of Observational Studies in Epidemiology (STROBE) providing recommendations to improve the quality of reporting of observational studies. (Vandenbroucke et al., 2007). Scientists searching for a communication venue may seek to gain credence and impact in medical journals or post preprints (public server online postings before peer review). This action may prevent haste in being the first one to publish a study.

Research findings are generally deemed credible when published by peer-reviewed scientific journals, government health agencies, and reputable medical organizations. A study's strength depends upon its size and well-designed clinical trials to decrease bias. Large sample sizes are seen as enhancing the reliability of p-values and investigative conclusions. However, research on some rare diseases may yield fewer sample sizes. A self-controlled case study research design (where subjects are their control) may be considered.

Clinicians confide in studies that helped create evidence-based guidelines (EBG) for clinical decision-making and standardized care. However, new or delayed studies may undermine a published study by providing contradictory or approximate truths. Peer-review is seen as enhancing the credibility of an author's paper. However, since some research articles suggest irregularities such as bias and fraud have occurred, peer-reviewed articles have come under scrutiny. (Reganault et al., 2018). Then, some researchers question if this metric provides proof or is a magnitude of error driving medical practice. Is it possible that reliance on such a metric could lead to unintended consequences in patient care? Is assessing the strength of evidence enough to rely upon if data is not transparent? As medical professionals strive for precision, they must balance statistical data with clinical judgment to ensure the best outcomes for their patients. Can medical practitioners identify which published journal articles are bias-free?

Some scientists have questioned the reliability of the current peer-review process and survey bias. The board of a professional organization asked an editor who expressed transparency concerns to step down. This situation arose because the underlying data cited in an author's paper was not made publicly available for review. Other peer reviewers identified the same concern. The group contends that authors were not obligated to share their underlying research data. Has such a review method ever influenced professional practice standards or guided personal health decisions? A Peer Reviewers' Openness Initiative was launched in 2017 to support openness and transparency in scientific research results. This action resulted in all scientists invested within the organization signing a pledge to follow transparency guidelines in the peer-review process. Do all peer reviewers embrace this initiative? Recognizing the above issues, the Center for Scientific Review (CSR) addresses bias and offers mitigation training for researchers and peer reviewers. (CSR, 2023).

Extant biases create significant challenges for clinical guideline organizations in interpreting, developing, and issuing professional recommendations. How can the affirmation of transparency be confidently accepted? The Grading of Recommendations Assessment, Development, and Evaluation (GRADE) system helps in judging "the certainty of evidence and strength of recommendations." (Murray et al., 20 23). Gaps in assessing the quality of studies in systematic reviews can affect decision-making therefore, trusted guidelines like the PRISMA statement are recommended. (Shaheen et al., 2023). Systematic reviews consolidating findings to address particular subject research questions may not contain the most current results. (Mickenautsch, 2010). As scoping reviews constantly change, using PRISMA-ScR along with other methodological guidelines has improved them. (Peters et al., 2021).

Research translation centers in the U.K., United States (U.S.), and Australia have been tasked with expediently reviewing new information for translation to healthcare and educational institutions. In Australia, strategies were studied to enhance real-world research translation however, not the translation and mobilization of knowledge for international education. (Edelman et al., 2020). Revising the framework criteria guiding translation decisions may help strengthen the translation process. (Wende et al., 2022). Excluding open and transparent studies on natural products diverts this consumer interest elsewhere. Furthermore, constant updating is required since decades pass between discoveries and the overturning of previous knowledge. Can those seeking healing now wait for what is considered absolute proof? Does this authenticity even exist when researchers advise that further research is needed to ardently support their conclusions? Investigators' perceptions and values may inadvertently skew findings or evidence affecting conclusions.

A former U.S. government agency official expressed concern about which interpreter's beliefs will finalize essential guidelines. As research evidence differs from infallible proof, there can be no credible one-care recommendations. This is of concern if the many biases influence conclusions established as evidence. How can bias be overridden if perspectives, beliefs, and values are automatic brain processes leading to perception bias (unconscious influence)? Partiality extends to all portions of the research process and to all persons involved. In blind clinical trials, data analysis can be exaggerated or framed to favor trial sponsors. Double-blind experiments with RCT may or may not limit these issues. Resolving issues necessitates a deeper understanding of the problem. Consciously aligning with the purpose, mission, and vision of a scientific experiment can contribute to the generation of genuine results.

Whether conscious or unconscious, COI produces bias and can intentionally change perceptions, as subjective study conclusions are rewarded in many ways. Generally, authors are to declare any COI, though do peer reviewers, journal editors, scientific translators, professional organizations, and policymakers declaring it? Even with a declared conflict of interest, research papers may lack objectivity or exhibit bias if they primarily portray emotions, opinions, or a negative perspective. To reduce bias, research enterprises may consider including incentives to decrease distorted conclusions. One motivating factor in untainted research may be recognizing "the best unbiased preclinical trial plan." (Huang et al., 2020).

To maintain research integrity and promote responsible investigative science, the core values and beliefs of scientists are significant. The fundamental principles of scientists conducting experiments play a crucial role in guiding ethical decision-making, promoting transparency, and ensuring that research is carried out with consideration for both the scientific community and society. Can an objective assessment commence if investigators are influenced by previous same-subject results, potentially inviting the same biases? Major journal editors have raised concerns about published clinical research and guidelines due to conflicts of interest (COI) that suggest various types of biases. Will respective professional associations investigate and consider these journal editors' and research investigators' concerns? Are certain industries or funding sources advocating for specific diagnoses and research that connect unexplained symptoms with existing or potential treatments? Are readers reviewing data with confirmation bias by looking for certain studies to favor established beliefs or contrasting them with disparate findings?

Do healthcare professionals have time to review all known study issues, including limitations and possible flawed study designs? While considering all aspects of a research study, federal agency medical and research information is publicly available online or can be requested from the Freedom of Information Act (available in many countries). So, how is the quality of research criteria reconciled within the international community?

For decades, universal guidelines for conducting ethical clinical trials did not exist. As testing on human beings occurred without consent but with indiscretion during multi-government experiments, an international consensus regarding human subjects became compulsory. The International Compilation of Human Standards, 2022, cites over 1,000 human protection standards for international organizations in

133 countries. Avoiding COI is essential for maintaining human study participants and research integrity. Is COI declared in regulatory agencies and policy regulators when reviewing research transparency? The United Nations Educational, Scientific, and Cultural Organization (UNESCO) uses the Recommendation for Science and Scientific Researchers. Member States help international research efforts under the standards of open science practices for transparency. They invite scientists to view research as a service. This perception can be the first step before the commencement of any investigative process. What regulations are in place to protect animal subjects in research?

Although organizations like the Animal Welfare Act, Public Health Service, and Association for Assessment and Accreditation of Laboratory Animal Care International exist, ethical concerns about animal subjects continue. These concerns include the suffering of sentient animals during and after testing, observing or hearing experiments conducted on other animals, and witnessing their eventual destruction. (Akhtar, 2015). Animals perceiving information through electromagnetic fields can predict when earthquakes or weather conditions are coming and act accordingly. Some marine animals use echolocation, which some blind persons have also experienced.

Does preclinical animal testing and results always translate to benefiting human beings? Although human and some animal genomes are similar, the genetic matchup is not 100%, thus, results can be skewed. "Finding antidotes should not compromise animal and then human safety." (Yang et al., 2021). Ethical concerns have led to offering the choice of using non-animal testing such as computer models, mathematical models, (Domínguez-Oliva et al., 2023) and volunteer human cells. However, animal studies are also subject to the same biases and COI encountered in human studies.

At the end of all study articles, journals could consider specifying if they followed the Center for Open Science, Open

Science Collaboration, TOP Guidelines, TOP factors, ICMJE recommendations, and COI declarations.

## How can these issues be resolved?

Despite known issues encountered within the research enterprise, it can have a promising future (chapter 9). All positive influences instituted now benefit the ends of biomedical research and its knowledge quality. Medical advancement requires diverse perspectives, vision, and fidelity to improve education, practice, and ultimately, human lives. Everyone involved in the process and fully committed to service and meticulous research practices helps meet these intended goals. This starts with a different way of thinking influencing perception.

"The task is not to see what has never been seen before, but to think what has never been thought before about what you see every day." (Erwin Schrödinger).

Curiosity (the willingness to ask questions without preconceived expectations) promotes the pursuit of truth and knowledge that impacts clinical practice. Biomedical researchers can perceive beyond limitations by critically assessing and perfecting every step of the investigative process. Being conscious of every way to transcend all biases, including research bias, leads to more impartial investigations and long-term solutions. Physicians can make a difference by perceiving beyond their own limitations and those of other medical professionals by presenting their own vision for clinical advancement. Before incorporating new findings into clinical practice, medical practitioners can achieve consensus by vetting the criteria for establishing evidence.

Perfecting the process establishing evidence for practice supports clinical actions, medical ethics, lobbying efforts, and allows for correct investigation of disease suspects to potentially resolve chronic conditions (chapter 6). By ensuring that evidence-based guidelines are both accurate and reliable, the scientific community can better serve the needs of society while maintaining the integrity of its work. Then licensed practitioners can confidently present correct findings to patients, to peers in symposiums, professional associations, and online medical forums.

When reviewing a paper's funding and COI statement, a reviewer can interpret if any financial or business ties during the research may constitute potential COI. As well, measuring patterns in scientific knowledge through scientometrics helps objectively determine their current and future relevance. Higher perspectives expand vision and fidelity to improve education, practice, and ultimately, human lives.

Medical providers can support researchers to address challenges within the scientific research field. Healthcare professionals and scientific investigators can encourage more independent research and funding of studies that explore the root causes of chronic diseases, lifestyle medicine, and other holistic approaches. They can promote open access to transparent research articles to make scientific findings available to doctors, other clinicians, researchers, and the public. Practitioners can urge their professional organizations to promote improved study designs that prioritize long-term, real-world outcomes rather than just short-term solutions. When medical professionals look beyond existing standard therapies and explore root-cause medicine, they can effectively address chronic disease states. A medical model centered around shared decisions derived from limited options cannot sustain itself. When a shortage of viable options limits a healthcare approach that relies on collaborative decision-making, it loses its effectiveness. As healthcare demands increase, these challenges limit patient autonomy and satisfaction. Addressing the challenges of sustainability in healthcare is essential for creating an environment that meets current needs and anticipates future demands. This proactive approach can ultimately shift the focus from merely managing symptoms to achieving true disease resolution, significantly enhancing healthcare delivery

Funders of government-sponsored, independent, and academic research studies can consider investing in a whole systems studies research approach. These studies utilize various methodologies, including pragmatic trials and mixed methods research. These research methods examine the interconnectedness of the human system within multiple areas of health for a multifaceted approach of identifying and addressing root causes of disease.

Medical professionals can consider becoming a researcher to help bridge gaps between biomedical studies and practice. Physicians can enroll and graduate from a combined M.D. and Ph.D. program to be a physician-scientist. Nurses with a Bachelor of Science Degree in Nursing can enter and graduate from a Master of Science in Nursing research program. All researchers can imagine how people will live based on their discoveries. Visualization (when one can see something as a reality) and holographic thinking (seeing all dimensions simultaneously) favor perceiving the impossible as viable.

As Chapter 4 examines the genesis of inimical job-related issues, clinicians can review the resources required to continue working fluently in human-centered environments. These resources include online professional support, specific tools, and perspectives that enhance communication and collaboration among team members. By fostering a positive workplace culture, clinicians can effectively address and mitigate the challenges they face to prevent harm.

# Chapter 4

## Overcoming Workplace Challenges

**"Choose a job you love and you'll never have to work a day in your life." ~ Confucius**

**"There's been a quantum leap technologically in our age, but unless there's another quantum leap in human relations, unless we learn to live in a new way towards one another, there will be a catastrophe." ~ Albert Einstein**

**"Be the change you wish to see in the world."**
**~ Mahatma Gandi**

**"Either you run the day or the day runs you." ~ Jim Rohn**

Every time the supervisor summoned nurses to their office, we observed a dysfunctional leadership style. Instead of receiving constructive guidance, condescending statements left us feeling intimidated. Rather than being written off the schedule, our manager scheduled this per diem nurse full-time for six months; then, with visible revelry, dismissed her in a meeting with Human Resources (HR). Was this action intended to serve as an example to the full-time nurses continuing to experience the same infringements? The act of repeatedly allowing unprofessional behavior in any healthcare setting is counterintuitive. Conceptually, a unified purpose in nursing realizes quality care. Did this leader's conduct result from self-projection, their perception of power, or job antipathy? The decision to weaken the team-leadership nexus has known consequences for any organization. Do healthcare facilities require behavioral science (health psychologist) and social science (social worker) professionals to audit organizational culture?

Behavioral and social science factors intersect with health and healing. These sciences appreciate preventing, predicting, and treating illness by addressing psychological dimensions affecting the body. They can also help formulate guidelines to fortify workplace culture for optimal health care delivery. After filing a complaint, the HR department could have enforced its own policies to render them meaningful. Perhaps like the nursing staff, they found it difficult to believe that a nursing leader could be a bully.

Bullying in the healthcare workplace setting is an overarching problem undermining facility purpose and objectives, potentially leading to employee and patient harm. The initial chain of reporting concerns starts with notifying one's supervisor. However, in this case, nurses were in the predicament of vertical harassment. Managerial compromise impeded the workflow, service, and intentions of the company's mission and vision statements. Although HR launched an investigation, other nurses remained mum for fear of reprisal. Post-investigation, HR continued supporting the supervisor (allowing violations to continue). Nurses were able to work without duress when HR passively supported nursing staff by eliminating that supervisory position, which eliminated the same position for another nurse at their sister hospital. Eventually, being in my truth and living beyond forgiveness (chapter 8) renewed personal power. This incident contrasted with my experiences with previous supportive nurse managers. I was curious about the above supervisor's self-perception. This type of behavior did not convey self-love, self-esteem, self-confidence, or self-respect. So, how can practitioners prevent such adverse experiences in the professional workplace?

Hospital administrators, Directors of Nursing (DON), and HR departments can proactively respect workers and patients when leading by example. They can frequently and maintain objectivity when meeting with staff, maintain an open-door policy, coordinate classes to help their team effectively communicate and collaborate, and honor their established policies. The following agencies are listed to help clinicians and certified nursing assistants (CNAs) handle workplace bullying and reprisal. Clinicians can consult their respective professional associations for guidance. The American Nurses

Association (ANA), American Medical Association (AMA), World Medical Association (physicians), World Health Professions Alliance, the U.S. Government, and the Joint Commission have guidelines to prevent and contend with bullying.

Due to the frequent intimidation, harassment, disruption, and threats, the workplace bullying we experienced appears to fit workplace violence (WPV) criteria. WPV also encompasses verbal abuse, physical assault, and homicide that affects employees, clients, vendors, and visitors according to the Occupational Safety and Health Administration. (OSHA). Employees can request the facility's bullying and WPV prevention and response program from HR if orientation does not cover these policies. The above safety recommendations include that employers adopt a zero-tolerance policy toward WPV and bullying to protect everyone in the workplace. However, policies are most effective when they are enforced.

Workplace violence is not limited to any one country. (Bernardes et al., 2021). Each year, violence in hospital settings cause a variety of personal and professional conflict issues. While some facilities post the actions that qualify as violence, it still occurs. Whether verbal, written, or carried out, there is a duty to report all incidences to a direct supervisor, administrator, and, potentially, law enforcement. Disparaging remarks and unacceptable behaviors by those in authority demean personal and facility values. Workplace bullying increases the risk of suicidal ideation. (Leach et al., 2020). Professional associations, state laws, the Joint Commission, and OSHA offer WPV prevention standards. CNAs can access their CAN association website.

Working under duress can catalyze symptoms, decrease performance, and increase the chance of mistakes or accidents. Many researchers find that the increased stress from WPV can lead workers to experience new medical conditions, exacerbate current ones, or contemplate or commit suicide. Top performers may face passive-aggressive hostility from leaders or team members due to perceived competition. Leadership cooperation in prevention and mitigation is compulsory, though hospital politics may hold a different agenda. Hospital boards, HR, the DON, and hospital administrators have the responsibility to set a positive example and live the facility's purpose and values to promote quality care. Those who choose to eschew policy are supporting breakdowns in system processes instead of facilitating potentially preventable adverse events. Support of bullying and WPV through allowance leads to co-opting a hostile working environment with consequences. Accidents and professional errors may arise, resulting in patient harm and employees fearing work. Several nurses have come to work only to discover that one or more employees had called off and were not replaced. A skeleton crew increases employee and patient burdens.

Many researchers deem medical and surgical residents working 24-hour shifts or more as unsafe. (Wong et al., 2020); thus, hospitals can opt to reevaluate this policy. In one facility, "back-to-back" scheduling was standard. When an employee's shift ended at 11:30 PM, it resumed at 7:00 AM the next day (even if nurses did not leave on time). This sometimes occurred during a scheduled ten-day stretch. Although we had more days off, working exhausted and sometimes understaffed did not benefit service. Attempting to support professional oaths and facility value statements seemed deceptive. Leadership advised nurses to avoid telling patients we were short-staffed. However, they failed to account for their awareness of staffing issues, the demands of shift work, and backbiting (judgments) influencing workplace direction.

In one hospital, there was a collaborative effort among staff. A high energy fluctuation infiltrated the intensive care unit, especially at night. The indirect calorimetry for our ventilated patients was met, but the nurses' energy and oxygen requirements were not. After midnight, while wolfing my meal down at the nurse's desk, a monitor displaying ventricular tachycardia required immediate action. We called a code blue and rushed the crash cart into this patient's room. He initially resisted the code team's response, rising out of bed and becoming combative. We saw the impossible occur as a patient in this arrhythmia fought against being coded. Unfortunately, this patient did not respond to resuscitation efforts, devastating everyone.

As nurses, we want to meet patient needs by always being available. However, to be of good service, taking scheduled breaks and mealtimes away from workstations is crucial to nourishment, energy, and renewal. As well, professionals require adequate sleep and rest before a scheduled shift. An impact on circadian rhythms includes night shift work can lead to sleep disturbances. Adequate sleep enhances cognitive and normal biological functioning and lowers chronic disease risks (Desai et al., 2024) The circadian rhythm (internal clock) disrupts homeostasis and can contribute to type 2 diabetes. (Tran et al., 2024). Jeffrey C. Hall, Michael Rosbash, and Michael W. Young won the Nobel Prize in chronobiology for identifying molecular mechanisms controlling the natural biological clock. They found rhythm disturbances affect humans, animals, and plants, producing changes due to a discrepancy between external and internal environments. These physical and psychological stressors predispose medical workers to psychological disorders, new diseases, or the worsening of current ones. (Yaribeygi et al., 2017). It changes glucoregulatory pathways, which can lead to pre-diabetes and diabetes. (Adamsson et al., 2018).

Disruptions in the sleep-wake cycle my hold the potential for medication and other medical milieu errors. Employers can consider this phenomenon when hiring, preparing work schedules, and with employees experiencing difficulties in shift work. Burnout is a preventable occupational hazard can indicate a lack of employer commitment. (Edú-Valsania et al., 2022). The disproportionate balance between work and personal life can result in difficulty coping and depersonalization. (Schalinski et al., 2015). Employers can outline and institute preventative measures (below) before burnout occurs to improve staff work life (sometimes considered an addendum to the triple aim framework). Lack of communication and staff support underpins stress manifesting as headaches, gastrointestinal symptoms, chest pain, or an exhaustion disorder. (Adamsson et al., 2018). Medical providers assessing stress can consider emotional factors as potential constituents of the energy of a symptom (chapter 6). With symptoms, employees call in sick, request leaves of absence, or show low productivity, leading to disciplinary action and attrition. Remediation efforts for these preventable situations include consulting one's medical and mental healthcare provider(s).

Many use the Employee Assistance Program (EAP) or other mental health providers after issues become overwhelming and unbearable. Leaders can be proactive to prevent the build-up of stressors and their aftermath. Employers can frequently connect with and assess workers and their workplace and follow up accordingly. They can provide stress management classes to help diffuse pressures and enhance work focus. Risk assessments and burnout tools can be provided so employees can assess and evaluate their responses. Healthcare workers may feel unable to air grievances with leadership in meetings for fear of reprisal. Recourse then reverts to expressing concerns and presenting consistent documentation to whom they report and an objective HR department.

In one facility, an issue presented that the hospital board, hospital administrator, and HR department required help to handle. The first task decided by a new DON was to reduce the salaries of all the nurses. While fellow employees thought the facility was in dire straits, the DON simultaneously authorized it to become a plush environment. This action caused dissatisfaction and squarely placed a financial burden upon the staff. As a group, we advocated for restoration of our wages and a better work environment to no avail. Some nurses yielded to the compounding issues of pay cuts and workload stress, while others sought employment elsewhere. When the physicians finally cleared the toxic work environment, stress had already caused physical harm to many of the nursing staff.

As personal and professional psychological and emotional duress intensifies, stress can become a silent killer (Yaribeygi et al., 2017). Walter Bradford Cannon suggests that brain systems are involved in the fight-or-flight response to a perceived threat and at times, the body is unable to adapt to the physical or emotional demand. (Godoy et al., 2018). The SHUT-D interview assesses susceptibility in dissociation to traumatic stress exposure. "Based on the psychobiological model of the defense cascade," shutdown dissociation from multiple traumatic stressors is increased. (Schalinski et al., 2015). Thus, emotional responses can trigger physiological reactions.

Stress and fear can increase work-related errors, accidents, and suicide. Employers can respond before it reaches the point where someone either attempts or commits suicide. In meetings, they can educate all employees to be aware of symptoms of depression and the services offered or that are accessible to them. Assistance and prevention measures can include employees having access to 24/7 onsite and telehealth crisis counseling. This service may have potentially saved one nurse's life. One December morning, during the handoff to me, it was unknown that a nurse had taken equipment and medication for home suicide. No one else had observed any unusual behavior prior to this day, during his 12-hour night shift, or that morning. The next day, his roommate notified our nursing supervisor that he had used Pavulon to take his life. It is unknown if things would have been different if mental health assistance had been available on-site.

Nurses divert patient supplies and medications for a variety of reasons. In two medical facilities, there were known narcotic discrepancies. The alleged drug diverters were good at concealing the misuse of these controlled substances (professional misconduct). Both cases allowed the facility-identified drug-addicted licensed nurses to voluntarily enter a rehabilitation program. Some U.S. states recognizing workers diagnosed with drug and alcohol addiction don't press charges if employees agree to enter recovery programs. Nurses can check their state laws or state Nurse Practice Act for guidance reporting. Patients have a right to receive the prescriptions they may rely on and pay for, and everyone deserves to be in a safe care environment. Each facility can address its policies and services offered in orientation classes and employee manuals. The National Alliance on Mental Health is a mental health resource for healthcare professionals. (www.nami.org).

The Suicide and Crisis Lifeline phone number is 988 in the United States (U.S.). One can check their country's designated mental health crisis phone number, which likely differs from the U.S. one. Many addiction rehabilitation efforts are integral in identifying and addressing an individual's underlying determinants behind their addictions. As they view each person as a whole being, they may reach those that may have with addiction and mental illness. Clinicians and health workers are required to navigate many other medical workplace issues that can affect their health.

All healthcare workers are subject to biological hazards. During orientation, I taught instruction on personal protective equipment (PPE) for those working in infection control and prevention. Is the breadth of this protection met if stress or other workplace issues distract workers from performing proper PPE techniques? Healthcare workers are concerned about exposure to job-related radiation. Those of us who have worked in a medical facility were given a device to measure occupational radiation exposure (high-energy beta, gamma, or X-rays). The absorbed radiation energy is taken up by body tissues and damages cells. Ionizing radiation reactive oxygen species (ROS) trigger DNA damage activating diseases, including cancer. (CDC, 2021). Medical facility employers are responsible for covering education regarding radiation exposure and protection programs in orientation. Additionally, they are responsible for establishing and maintaining a dosimetry program, overseeing radiation protection policies and procedures, and conducting internal audits. (OSHA). Workers can request their confidential occupational radiation dosimetry report from their employer.

Most employees are led to believe that low levels of ionizing radiation from diagnostics are not harmful. However, one must consider the repeated cumulative or lifetime effects of all types of personal and professional exposures. Repeated CT scans and radiation exposure increase cancer risks. (Cao et al., 2022). The Environmental Protection Agency (EPA) offers a calculation tool for professionals to estimate radiation dosage from all types of exposures. (EPA, 2022). Other personal risk factors include:

- Natural radiation (radon, cosmic rays)
- Airport X-Ray systems (luggage, shoes, purses)
- Full-body scanning systems.

The EPA also factors in geographical regions, internal radiation from food and water, and weapons test fallout exposures. Moreover, there are concerns regarding the cumulative subjection to low radiation levels (cell phones, electrical towers, radio signals, and dental X-rays). The ongoing effects of the atomic bomb and the contamination from the Chernobyl and Fukushima fallouts are also a concern (EPA, 2022). You can consult your personal healthcare provider for guidance on these matters and to develop a potential plan for informed, shared decision-making.

Inpatient medical and outpatient centers are required to ensure a facility provides appropriate protective equipment for the type of work performed. This includes providing and having workers use lead shields, aprons, gloves, and glasses when appropriate. Radioprotectors (plants and herbs containing polyphenols) can increase antioxidation and scavenge free radicals (Jagetia, 2007). Patients and medical facility employees are exposed to chemical hazards from disinfectants, certain caustic medications, lab tissue fixatives, etc. Each facility must provide first aid procedures. (The National Institute for Occupational Safety and Health, NIOSH, 2018). Generally, chemical manufacturer safety data sheets advise workers to wash their hands after contact with any chemical and other hazardous substances (even after doffing gloves). Additionally, they should adhere to appropriate storage and disposal protocols for chemicals.

Since the 2020 pandemic, more medical professionals started working at home. Thus, prolonged sitting created a potential risk for the development of chronic medical conditions. It is prudent to have an ergonomically aligned workstation and chair. (OSHA). Some work safety organizations suggest standing/stretching every 2 hours and walking for at least 30 minutes (at lunchtime if able). And using variable workstations, comfortable footwear, and rubber mats for long periods of standing. An institution with a physical therapy department may be able to teach worker safety regarding lifting and other ergonomic techniques. Healthcare workers can visit the NIOSH website for their Lifting Equation or NLE Calc APP to calculate the overall risk index for manual lifting tasks. This application provides risk estimates that help evaluate lifting tasks to reduce the incidence of low back injury. Employers may offer home workers computer tutorials to prevent various ergonomic injuries.

Organizations generally encourage professional workers to take scheduled breaks and mealtimes away from on-site and home workstations. Prolonged sitting and eating quickly can cause issues for workers. In a study, various symptoms, including belching and acid reflux, were related to eating too fast, eating at irregular mealtimes, and consuming certain foods. (Li et al., 2020). High salt intake, Helicobacter pylori, and sodium nitrate in processed foods may be linked to chronic gastritis, which potentially may lead to cancer. (Li et al., 2020). All of these stressors and workplace issues combined with personal factors present the potential for poor performance and medication errors. Awareness of all issues may help strengthen healthcare policy and procedure (P&P), as medical workplaces have a duty to ensure employee and patient safety.

An in-house pharmacy is a resource for helping to create a facility's P&P and responding to any medication questions.

Unintended patient harm may be prevented by meticulously following a facility's medication administration P&P and asking questions "The only stupid question is the one that is never asked." (Ramon Bautista). Medical facility employers can be aware of issues caused by overworked and disrupted prescribers and medication administrators. Following the six rights of medication administration does not preclude sincerely questioning prescribers when there are concerns (chapter 5). Perceiving beyond, health workers suggesting corrective measures and envisioning how issues in medicine can be resolved help direct energy toward that reality (chapter 2).

Preventing discord in the workplace creates a conflict-free environment and encourages clinicians to act according to their professional codes. This enhances productivity, service delivery, and viewing a facility's vision and mission efforts as imaginable, enabling the facilitation of quality healthcare delivery. Compromised patients benefit from congenial and rested workers and deserve their full attention and expertise.

From an expanded perspective, clinicians can be aware of transparent biomedical research articles that offer a difference in improving the patient and provider experience (chapter 3). They can evaluate the level of commitment and enjoyment within their professional roles and make decisions accordingly. Each clinician can assess if they are going to a routine job or if they have enthusiasm about doing everything possible to heal the sick.

As professionals across various disciplines unite their expertise, they create a robust network that addresses systemic issues and improves outcomes for patients. Ultimately, embracing collaboration is not merely advantageous; it is essential for evolving the healthcare system into one that prioritizes collective effort and shared success. When all medical employees and leadership work to prevent and resolve identified issues, compassion is renewed.

The coming chapters continue to outline clinician and patient empowerment within the clinical setting. Chapter 5 emphasizes understanding and respecting individual client perspectives that establish personal truth creating choices. As medical workers gain clarity on the goal of medicine, both caregivers and medical consumers can perceive the authenticity of medical care. This mutual understanding fosters a more collaborative relationship between clinicians and patients, ultimately enhancing the quality of care. By prioritizing transparency and respect for client perspectives, the healthcare system can better align with ethical standards and patient needs.

# Chapter 5

## Patient Perspectives of Healthcare Delivery

**"I attribute my success to this: I never gave or took an excuse."**
**~ Florence Nightingale**
**"The very first requirement in a hospital is that it should do**
**patients no harm." ~ Florence Nightingale**

**"Quality healthcare can also be defined as:" "Providing the right**
**healthcare services in a right way in the right place at the right**
**time by the right provider to the right individual for the right**
**price to get the right results." ~ Ali Mohammad Mosadeghrad**

Magnetic Resonance Imaging (MRI) studies have established neurobiological correlates creating neurological symptoms related to psychological outcomes in caregivers (Smagula & Aizenstein, 2023). Researchers found that perceived negative statements or words relating to discomfort intensified pain more than neutral or positive language (Brodhun et al., 2024). Entanglement between healer and client may be responsible for healing (Matos et al., 2021). The ability of collective perceptions can persist through the universe's quantum interactions. This interconnectedness suggests that our grasp of reality is shaped by both the microcosm of quantum phenomena and the macrocosm of collective human consciousness (chapter 10).

When care measures fail to elicit a desired response, mutual dissatisfaction can occur. As populations differ, treatments may not allow individualized attention due to heterogeneity (chapter 3). The placebo effect may meet the distinct needs of individuals across various populations. That is, it can tap into the psychological and emotional aspects of treatment, offering a tailored response that resonates with individual experiences. This phenomenon emphasizes the need to consider personal factors in medical care, even when standardized treatments are applied. There are "psycho-neuro-endocrine-immune mechanisms of the placebo effect." (Ortega et al., 2022). A real brain-body placebo effect is "caused by cognitive and emotional changes, expectation of symptom changes, or classical conditioning." (Beauvais, 2017). This may be interpreted as the manifestation of emotions (bottom-up processing) and sensory perception (top-down processing).

The above researchers' findings indicate that practitioner expectations can be the impetus for experiencing nocebo effect (Preface & Introduction). As just the perception of something can move that thought (energy) into being (chapter 8). Most patients have high expectancies of their prospective medical interventions. Patients who understand their conditions and are actively involved in their care, can make better decisions. (Waweru et al., 2015). As a clinician-patient, are underlying issues expressed in each complaint always heard, understood, and fully addressed? Is there a mutual understanding of managing symptoms or treating disease from its core for permanently correction (chapter 6)? Patients are increasingly expecting a cure to alleviate their medical conditions.

Many people have perceived and moved beyond their circumstances and diagnosed conditions (chapter 8). However, if examination and diagnostics fail to provide a precise diagnosis and interventions directed at the root cause, this reality can appear unattainable. This limits patient shared decision-making power in selecting the most perceived efficacious intervention(s). The Society to Improve Diagnosis in Medicine (Preface) aims to improve diagnosis and eliminate harm from diagnostic errors. Their collaboration has attracted many healthcare institutions to support accurate diagnosis and preventing harm.

As patients trust healthcare professionals to solve the underpinnings of symptoms that may cause suffering, are healthcare systems able to respond properly? Chapter 2 reviewed how patients can be influenced by those in positions of authority. Are medical systems promoting the acceptance of symptom management, precluding full investigation of common underlying causes (chapter 6)? If the answer involves the word impossible, then this level of perception will always generate that reality.

Joint Commission-accredited organizations must have assessment tools and procedures in place to deal with pain while considering whether the patient prefers pharmaceutical or nonpharmacological approaches. (Joint Commission, 2022). Despite the lack of a mandate to confirm the cause of pain, providers treat chronic idiopathic pain. Therefore, patients and providers continue to experience frustration as they struggle to understand the etiology of symptoms. However, some lifestyle providers consider using a more comprehensive assessment that includes evaluating emotional and mental factors associated with chronic pain.

In 2016, the United States (U.S.) Congress passed the 21st Century Cures Act to assist in faster medical product development for expeditious consumer use. Many may find advantages in new medical technology, devices, and products. Depending on their expectations, patients may believe that all available treatments are intended to be curative. Medical consumers want goods and services to target the underlying mechanisms of their diagnosed conditions. Healthcare providers are increasingly placed in a position where their charges are requesting that the perceived impossible become recognized as possible. This obliges healthcare providers to review the strengths and limitations of research guiding evidence-based medicine (EBM) (chapter 3).

Some providers see EBM akin to a cookbook approach, as algorithms direct complex decision-making, while others view it as a logical problem-solving mechanism. In either view, how can medicine precisely respond to medical information having a short "half-life" of scientific truth (chapter 3)? Will expedient translational review of disparate replicated transparent data close the gap between symptom management and cure? While the public awaits the years required to conduct private and government-sponsored clinical investigations, will there be complete relevance in that knowledge?

Clinicians must always follow the clinical ethics of **"autonomy, justice, beneficence, and nonmaleficence."** (Mousavi, 2024) in their interactions with patients. Violation of these obligations can constitute malfeasance. There is mutual disappointment when patients perceive continuing suffering by living with symptoms or unintended effects of provider-prescribed interventions. In personal interactions with patients, healing, or wholeness in the form of complete restoration (cure) is the expectation of one faction of the provider-patient relationship. **Patients and their sentient cellular structures (Baluška et al., 2021) seek solutions rather than simply being told there are no alternatives.** Every day, scientists are working to create solutions. Many biomedical researchers who overcame scientific investigative challenges seek recognition of their contrasting findings (all chapters) for appropriate application.

When patients express dissatisfaction with the medical product, they can feel helpless. If patients perceive their only options as defective, irreparable, and unreturnable, they can experience a sense of powerlessness. If persistent frustration creates a perception of continuing the same thing and expecting different results (Albert Einstein), then a conscious and responsive medical community is compulsory (chapter 9). Many licensed medical providers identify with patients' discontent with determinism and feel limited within current practice standards. Those viewing the healthcare delivery system as not fulfilling its intention and mission can respond.

When clinicians submit concerns to their respective professional associations, awareness exists. Following up brings personal and professional concerns one step closer to being recognized, understood, and addressed. Healthcare professionals can consider connecting with or founding patient advocate organizations and associations if there is inadequate or no response. Those passionate about benefiting medical consumers can consider forming a strong coalition that works together with like-minded people and organizations. Clinicians are encouraged to submit their concerns and ideas for discussion in professional and organizational forums. What are the risks versus benefits of inaction?

Patients looking for relief outside of established medical practices can trigger mutual frustration. Believing remedies for their ailments exist, the Internet and social media have been used to self-diagnose and treat. Others visit complementary practitioners and integrative care providers for a different outcome. Many believe addressing the interconnectedness of human components helps the body naturally respond. Then, consumers may perceive providers who focus on a single complaint (the affected body part) as practicing within a narrow scope. More and more people believe that healing can occur when all their bodily aspects are addressed. This includes having their spiritual connections recognized and addressed which prompts the development of these types of tools (Ghaderi et al., 2018). Many believe that self-realization and self-actualization (chapter 9) promotes and even assures natural healing.

The concept of the mind-body connection that has been around for centuries has garnered debate over the past decades (Preface). However, a gap is created when providers do not recognize its role in disease and healing thus, hindering correct diagnosis and interventions. As a result, physical symptoms are prioritized over psychological issues. "Interoceptive self-report scales have served as primary assessment tools in mind-body research." (Van Bael et al., 2023).

As well, there is no standard recognition of the complete evaluation of the perceived abstract (spiritual) feature and applying it to a psychological or medical condition. Some providers may consider multiple assessments cumbersome and without any perceived practical application. Some Australian and developed Eastern Asian nations' government-funded organizations recognize that unresolved trauma and emotions can catalyze ailments in or affecting specific body organs (chapter 6). Until there is a standardized conceptual framework recognizing the various factors affecting the human condition, they remain incognizant and unaddressed. Could people perceive this stance as an omission and a basis for legal action (chapter 9)? Disregarding factors that patients believe affect their health can drive them to search for perceived healing measures elsewhere. (Bozek et al., 2020).

Those diagnosed with multimorbidity have a higher use of complementary and alternative medicine (CAM). (CDC, 2016). The 2007 National Health Interview Survey found 38.2 percent of adults and 12 percent of children used CAM within 12 months of the survey. (NCCAM Strategic Plan 2011-2015). Due to increased interest in natural therapies worldwide and frustration with living with symptoms, CAM usage may be expected to rise. This may account for the launch of a five-year study to develop personalized nutritional recommendations. The Nutrition for Precision Health by the All of Us Research Program considers developing algorithms to predict individual responses to foods. (NIH, 2023). There has been a randomized control trials of tailored diets for type 2 diabetes individuals in Massachusetts, USA. And a ten-year (2020-2030) study (Strategic Plan for NIH Nutrition Research) to review food as medicine is underway.

According to the National Center for Complementary and Integrative Health (NCCIH), clinical investigations aim to evaluate CAM modalities in disease prevention, health maintenance, and symptom management. Can clinicians confidently examine the methodology (Chapter 3). Will conclusions coincide with other researchers' findings supporting the benefits of certain foods, spices, herbs, and other interventions specified throughout this text? Ancient cultures effectively used plant-derived compounds for pain relief and treatment of disease. Traditional knowledge still guides the use of some of these natural therapies, such as aspirin, artemisinin, and certain childhood cancer treatments. (WHO, 2023).

Sometimes, the field of medicine can seem generic. However, every unique person can exhibit contrasting symptoms, and because of differences in some biochemical responses or other variables, they may react differently to the same therapies. But trial and error attempts to discern unique nuances can cause harm and suffering. When my then-husband was diagnosed with chronic diarrhea, it took several months of eliminating medications before this symptom was finally diagnosed as a result of a prescribed medication side effect. Several friends and patients perceived as malingerers had to seek a second opinion for correct diagnoses. These situations raise the question, "How can medicine identify and address the root causes of disease instead of depending on automated responses?"

In our innocence as children, we continually asked people, "Why?" until receiving a perceived appropriate answer. The Toyota Motor Corporation manager, Taiichi Ohno, used the "Ask 'why' five times about every matter" approach to drill down to the root cause of every issue. Albert Einstein asserts that the answer lies in asking the correct question. "If I had an hour to solve a problem and my life depended on the solution, I would spend the first 55 minutes determining the proper question to ask, for once I know the proper question, I could solve the problem in less than five minutes." Can this level of complex problem-solving assist researchers in reaching root causes of disease and help providers with patients perceived as challenging, demanding, or chronic complainers? Labeling clients as difficult or, as with my friend Annie, arbitrarily dismissing symptoms as psychosomatic (medical gaslighting) hinders the diagnostic process (Preface & Introduction). This is inconsistent with the medical rubric, as many other patients have been sent away with unaddressed symptoms, which had progressed and cost them their lives.

To prevent missed diagnoses and assumptions, practitioners can consider reviewing diverse scientific research papers. To avoid incorrect diagnoses leading to erroneous or no intervention, "fitness brackets" may assist in reaching the correct determination; strategies "such as 2-step testing algorithms, including repeat testing, are used when prevalence is beyond the inherent limitations of any single test." (Olliaro & Torreele, 2021). Although molecular, serological, and antigen testing have improved, "combining serological methods with RT-PCR for SARS-CoV-2 detection" has demonstrated precise diagnosing. (Alamri et al., 2023). Authors point to this strategic method to prevent and control future outbreaks (Alamri et al., 2023). Attention to specific symptoms can lead to targeted testing (chapter 6) or specialist referrals that help doctors accurately diagnose medical conditions. Reviewing case studies may offer a tentative guideline for attending to people diagnosed with a rare medical condition.

Patients have raised concerns when hearing their provider say, "Continue doing whatever it is you are doing." When it is unknown what is effective for a patient, true evaluation of their interventions cannot be determined. Are there clear directions for patients to report something that may no longer work? Obtaining patient-expressed needs and preferences is followed by honoring their informed say. Professional organizations agree that patient input (shared decision-making) in care is a patient right (Shaghayegh et al., 2014). This observance disclaims the perception of provider-centered care. In attempting to deliver quality, is the patient focused on rehabilitative, comfort, or curative measures? Understanding an individual's healing perspective projects practitioners toward an individualized patient-preferred course of care. However, can cure realistically be a viable medical goal? Providers seeing desperate patients wanting what is putatively beyond the perceived capacity of medical care will always generate that reality. Providers stating that probability, the odds, and limitations as truth present challenges in overcoming them. A friend diagnosed with cancer doesn't know if they can beat the odds. Clinicians can be sensitive to patients' distresses by choosing openness through objectivity and non-judgment, be mindful of the nocebo effect, and investigate disparate scientific research articles to perceive beyond collectively established limits.

Providers are frustrated when patients experience harm from adverse effects. However, practitioners may perceive harm if they fail to initiate the standard recommendations for a particular diagnosis. Though, neither the patient nor the provider may be reporting adverse events or quality concerns of pharmacologic substances or biologics to the U.S. Food and Drug Administration (FDA). This is one way that scientists and healthcare practitioners can help to bridge the gap between ineffective care standards and patient expectations. Improvements in the scientific research construct (chapter 3) can help create a foundation for healing with a generable definition of health and disease states (chapter 1) and enhancement of correct pathology (chapter 6) for precise therapeutics. Does the current time allotted, along with a provider's past experiences and the scope of their medical education, allow for a comprehensive understanding of each patient?

In practice, limited interaction and communication issues can preclude the entire client perspective. This can hinder a patient's understanding of medical conditions, tests, and options. Confusion about the meaning and implications of symptoms can lead to a distorted perception. This could lead to despair if diagnostic opinions are viewed as a predetermined fate where no other possibility could exist. Patients continue expressing frustration in hearing common medical conditions are something they just must live with. Living within a medical system's limitations affirms ever being able to relieve symptoms or suffering; then, some patients have perceived the need to become their own advocates. Self-preservation is personal, as clinicians and patients who follow current standards of care experience the same burdens. Can we collectively continue accepting that there are no other options in certain medical situations?

That thought expressed as truth, has proven to be very powerful. Some people have prepared for their demise and imagined their future according to authoritative professional opinions a potential reaction to the nocebo effect, (Introduction & Chapter 1). What are the consequences if healthcare professionals fail to look beyond established limitations and continue to practice within their confines? This narrow focus may perpetuate health disparities and hinder the overall advancement of the healthcare delivery system. There is power in pursuing the truth, regardless of what it may be (chapters 3 & 6).

Nonverbal communication can be quite powerful. Such unintentional actions can influence another's perceptions and their decisions regarding care. Healthcare staff may be unaware of their behavior due to automatic and unconscious mental processes and work-related issues (chapter 4). Attention and focus on present endeavors devoid of needless conflict meet the basic consideration of service. Disharmony in a care environment can preclude healthcare workers from anticipating and fulfilling client needs. The healing efforts of others can depend on the reconciliation of caregiver attitudes, judgments, and perspectives. This cultivates relationships and builds trust in human-centered care environments. The actions, attitudes, and errors of one employee can and have eroded confidence in the entire facility and medical system.

Behavioral and social science principles in psychology and sociology provide a conceptual framework for understanding perceptions and responses. Theoretical models such as the health belief model have been applied to health measures. When patients are not compliant with their provider's orders, clinicians wonder if they take their condition seriously. However, this scenario allows clinicians to assess and address a broader range of a patient's concerns by understanding why an individual does not perceive benefits. Has the provider ascertained if their patient feels they don't have time to care for their own conditions as they focus on caring for another?

Conflict with providers can develop if a patient's distress arises as an experience of harm from appraised guidelines. These practice standards, partially regarding systematic reviews can imply that risks are too significant if they are not used. This direction has superseded the right of patient input and informed refusal, often putting uniformity before individual freedoms. One patient reported that their physician insisted they stop a generally deemed safe, natural product yielding normal cholesterol results and start a standard guideline. This patient reluctantly complied, not realizing their right to shared decision-making. Despite informing their physician about the adverse effects of the prescribed regimen, they received instructions to persist with it, which may have potentially constituted malfeasance (causing harm).

Medical providers did not administer a depression screening inventory or questionnaire to several of my senior patients who lost their spouses. Seeming to fit uncomplicated bereavement, they initially declined mood-altering interventions. However, they reluctantly submitted to authority. Their providers did not ascertain the underlying factors of their emotional pain. Were they also missing their spouse because of financial or physical assistance, the only current form of love or companionship, feeling multiple losses at once, etc.? Therefore, it is possible that their depression may not have been resolved as the underlying factor(s) were not recognized or addressed. These patients were surprised that they didn't receive a referral to a mental health provider (under the collaborative care model). Unfulfillment of the Triple Aim goals left these clients without perceptible value from their interactions, leading to wanting to switch medical providers.

When medical providers don't include but ignore a patient's preferences, they violate the medical ethics of autonomy, which can constitute impropriety. Can perceptual positioning (seeing things from another's vantage point) lead to a deeper understanding of patient beliefs? Clinicians can dismiss automatic value judgments to gain appreciation of another's perception while not adopting their point of view (Yuan et al., 2017). However, practitioners may unintentionally use to persuade clients of perceived limits (nocebo) and press agendas. Unshared decisions can lead to helplessness, frustration, and harm, potentially resulting in liability. People then may consult the Internet or others, thus missing interactive lifestyle teaching.

Providers can consider working with each patient to map out a precise individual interventional care plan that meets the person's beliefs and perceptions of healing. Working together toward common goals benefits the healthcare delivery system by creating a palpable culture of caring. The development of an individualized care plan exemplifies a transformative approach in healthcare, where collaboration between providers and patients is at the forefront. By engaging patients in the planning process, healthcare providers ensure that the interventions not only address medical needs but also resonate with the individual's beliefs and perceptions of healing. This can include assessing their cultural and personal beliefs about disease, healing, and health maintenance. Instead of hearing and internalizing a disease as incurable, biological responses may be influenced if a perception reflects personal belief that their body has the power to heal, or other cognitive restructuring that challenges recurrent negative thought patterns. Practitioners may be reluctant to provide what they believe as false hope, however, researchers cited within this text provide insight as to how belief can create reality.

There has been a multitude of hospital complaints lodged by patients and families. Medical institutions are required to have internal processes to address these and all other types of complaints. Even when prevention processes are in place, human error can occur. Upon arriving at the hospital, my then-husband advised he was given a bag of intravenous fluid (IV) during the night. He became one of the thousands of people that year experiencing preventable harm. The doctor had automatically employed a set of checklist protocols, and the nurse precipitously followed the written orders. As a volume prescription, IV fluid is subject to the same tenets of medication administration. Despite adhering to the six rights of medication administration, the prescriber should have questioned the order before proceeding. Professionals cannot automatically follow predesigned directions if there are any questions or doubts. In this case, the nurse omitted to ask the physician if this patient with only one kidney that was not producing urine (diagnosed at that facility as due to obstruction) should receive IV fluid. Since the fluid could not be excreted, he developed respiratory distress.

The risk manager promptly received a written grievance about this preventable harmful experience. A root cause analysis would attempt to enhance process improvement strategies to prevent a future sentinel event. Did the above error stem from a communication issue or perceived hierarchical doctor-nurse relationship? Or were night shift employees experiencing cognitive impairment due to being overworked, exhausted, short-staffed, or sleep issues (circadian rhythm disturbances) (chapter 4)?

Many patients and families feel betrayed by a preventable medication error, misdiagnosis, and delay in diagnosis resulting in intervention lags that can contribute to harm. A patient questioning a therapy can serve as a red flag and alert a practitioner to double-check or challenge their orders. This action may avert the commission of a medication or other error. Mistakes and omissions have led many patients to view their medical providers as still practicing. Investigating a model like Ulric Neisser's (chapter 2) for potential application in healthcare delivery may prevent incorrect decisions leading to clinical errors. As researchers explain how beliefs and perceptions yield personal and collective reality (chapter 2), the medical community may see how it can influence behavior, interactions, and decisions in medical practice.

Errors that don't cause harm and near misses should still be reported to the organization and FDA.gov to identify and correct the underlying causes of an error. Some research organizations estimate that each year, nearly 100,000 inpatients die due to preventable medical errors. Medical errors are the third leading cause of death (**Atanasov et al., 2020**), though it is not recognized as a determination on death certificates. Currently, this documentation defaults to an International Classification of Disease (ICD) code to which errors of omission and commission are not assigned.

Perceiving beyond, clinicians can assess the accuracy of patient satisfaction surveys. Consumers may be responding to being satisfied with clinician caring rather than the actual value found in the healing they received. Organizations attempt to learn about patients' perspectives of their hospital experience from the Hospital Consumer Assessment of Healthcare Providers and Systems (HCAHPS). This survey allows insight into what patients believe is important to improve care quality. However, are survey questions routine or misinterpreted by medical consumers? If patient feedback is consistent with dissatisfaction with diagnosis or cure, will healthcare facilities designate a multi-professional and medical consumer board to review diverse scientific evidence? If physicians and nurses adequately identify the gaps between research and practice (chapter 3), will institutions be readily amenable to recommended changes for expedient implementation?

There are clear guidelines for referring patients to a specialist, but not for the patients with chronic disease who may be consistently unresponsive to standards of care. How can providers choose interventions to target conditions if they don't identify their root cause? Government agencies, professional associations, and guideline developers understanding research challenges can review the most non-biased, transparent research conclusions to avoid someone doing harm. Chapter 6 explores the etiology of underlying disease mechanisms to evaluate a solid foundation for healing. A comprehensive understanding of disease pathology is essential in delivering precise medical care. Many researchers associate a viral suspect with some cancers, neurological disorders, and other diseases (Serafini et al., 2019). If a clinical trial started to test a vaccine (NIH, 2022) against a virus, will medical providers confront this pathogen at the viral level?

Persistent curiosity may prevent medical providers from solely attributing lifestyle to some chronic diseases. Providers seeking a deeper understanding of disease mechanisms and healing perspectives strengthen healthcare delivery.

# Chapter 6

## Constituents of Disease Pathology

**"It is far more important to know what person the disease has than what disease the person has."** ~ Hippocrates

**"We are not human beings having a spiritual experience. We are spiritual beings having a human experience"**
**~ Pierre Teilhard de Chardin**

"It isn't that they cannot find the solution. It is that they cannot see the problem." ~ G.K. Chesterton

"We fail more often because we solve the wrong problem than because we get the wrong solution to the right problem."
~ Russell L. Ackoff

Yet another patient inquired about the cause of his new illness and then asked, "Why do bad things happen to good people?" This belief seems to align with the perception that medical conditions are random events. Some patients attribute disease and suffering to determinism, a mathematical framework, or chance occurrences, rather than a mechanism of cause and effect. Consequently, if free will is perceived as an illusion, one may embrace fate over personal agency or metaphysical beliefs.

Based on education and experience, some licensed medical professionals have advised patients of the "odds" (Preface) or chance of surviving a certain diagnosis. They may intend this guidance to help patients understand the provider's opinion of their prognosis and make informed decisions about their affairs and treatment options. However, this belief can sometimes lead to misconceptions about the role of medical expertise in understanding health outcomes. Statistical terms often present the odds, potentially misleading patients who may view them as definitive predictions instead of possibilities.

The journey through chronic disease often reveals a profound struggle against the physical manifestations of illness and the quest for control over one's health and life. As patients contend with their medical circumstances, they frequently find themselves questioning the very origins of their afflictions, seeking answers that often seem elusive.

Many medical providers have informed patients that reversing certain disease states is not possible; instead, patients must learn to manage their conditions. Despite this collective belief presented as fact, many patients maintain that achieving relief from suffering through disease reversal is possible through lifestyle clinics and transparent research. This shared perception has intensified the commitment of numerous biomedical researchers and medical practitioners (Preface) to identify the underlying causes of symptoms to address them at their source.

Health challenges have long been the impetus for solving human burdens. Throughout time, imaginations have brought viable alternatives to fruition. Many documented accounts describe parents solving their child's rare disease origins and developing a treatment or cure. However, time constraints, resources, or acumen in such research efforts can default to limited choice, palliative care, or surrender. Laypeople establishing causations, treatments, and cures for rare diseases amplify the call for sophisticated medical systems and research sectors to resolve common chronic disease states.

Practitioners navigating the complex landscape of medical research data often reveals a troubling undercurrent. They fear facing reprisal when applying concordant but non-standardized research data. This apprehension stifles progress and leaves medical consumers feeling abandoned in their quest for effective therapeutic options. As individuals with chronic disease struggle with their health challenges, the need for comprehensive disease constituent identification becomes increasingly urgent. By asking practical questions that tackle this issue, a new perspective can help connect biomedical research and real-world use. The synthesis of assessing concerns and identifying solutions, paves the way for a more informed and supportive healthcare landscape. This call for comprehensive disease constituent identification highlights the need for a more nuanced understanding of health conditions to move beyond mere symptom relief. By addressing root causes of chronic conditions, informed providers can better meet the expectations of medical consumers seeking holistic care.

Medical practitioners and their professional organizations reviewing diverse biomedical research papers can narrow the gap between managing and targeting the underlying energy of a disease. Therefore, this chapter reviews researchers' conclusions about the multifactorial antecedents of disease affecting biological coherence. Their findings lead to a new perspective on the link between cause and effect and the creation of a better way to make clinical and shared patient-provider decisions.

Can medicine study the interconnectedness of human systems to provide a theoretical framework and a unified explanation for the development of chronic disease? Which model is more effective: the disease-based model (standardized treatment of symptoms) or the holistic-based model (recognizing the interconnections within the body)? Or would a hybrid model be more efficient for understanding disease for more personalized therapies?

The chain of infection components indicates the critical pathways through which infections can take hold and propagate. (NIOSH, 2022). However, in many non-communicable disease states, are all disease agents* consistently considered as potential underlying causes? Fully understanding these elements creates a multifaceted perspective that illustrates how various influences converge to contribute to the development and progression of chronic diseases. By identifying these underlying mechanisms, providers are better equipped to inform patients of prevention and therapeutic strategies.

Reviewing various models can clarify and harmonize the ontology of causal assessment (Shimonovich et al., 2021). Rothman's framework shows how different factors interact to determine causal agency. As not everyone exposed to an infectious agent develops a disease and engaging in a risk factor does not always cause illness, what supplies the foremost impulse for the development of a disease? Approaching this question holistically, complete patient data may guide pinpointing causal mechanisms. A comprehensive patient assessment prompts ordering targeted lab tests. (Fisher & Gupta, 2022). Specific testing may pinpoint *viral suspects, low levels of necessary metals or the toxicity of unnecessary heavy metals (HMs), other toxins, pathogens, and deficiencies. Experienced medical providers and mental health professionals may identify the effects of post-traumatic stress disorder (PTSD) and traumatic events in childhood (adverse childhood experiences or ACEs**) in disease pathology. Damaged cells resulting from the above overlooked influences can affect gene expression.

The evolving understanding of epigenetic factors has transformed providers' perception of disease causation, shifting the narrative from a strictly hereditary framework to one that acknowledges the significant role these modifications play in health and illness. Signaling pathways that affect transcription factors can become unbalanced, leading to the development of many diseases (Casamassimi et al., 2023). Proinflammatory pathways are associated with modulating chronic disease, including obesity. Adipose tissue releases adipokines, leading to inflammation (Kirichenko et al., 2022) the undercurrent of disease. Obesity is considered a balance between consumed caloric energy and the metabolic output of excess energy stored in fat cells (Lin & Li, 2021). However, what are the underlying the mechanisms involved?

The significance of emotions that increase cortisol from the adrenal glands (Knezevic et al., 2023) and the liver's role in insulin resistance and non-alcoholic fatty liver disease (NAFLD) (Wazir et al., 2023) may be disregarded. Many researchers find that ACEs** can influence emotional dysregulation, which may lead to obesity and other medical conditions affecting individuals from childhood into adulthood (page 90). When normal microbiota enzyme action is interrupted, bile acid changes make it easier for fat to be absorbed and weight gain to occur (Sarmiento-Andrade et al., 2022). When the gut microbiota responds to epigenetic changes with increased appetite, reducing caloric intake can reduce the likelihood of obesity (Lin & Li, 2021). Dysbiosis (from antibiotic usage) via the gut-brain axis can lead to autism (Taniya et al., 2022), obesity (Lin & Li, 2021), type 1 and type 2 diabetes, and gastrointestinal, immunologic, and neurocognitive conditions (Dahiya & Nigam, 2023).

"The field is now able to visualize, measure, and manipulate engram neurons with an impressive level of specificity, enabling the role and evolution of the engram to be understood across memory stages." (Guskjolen & Cembrowski, 2023). Can fat cell and body organ memory engrams activate or reactivate disease as someone relives a traumatic experience? Is the activation of negative engram memories contributing to the ongoing cycle of symptoms and the lack of response to some therapies? Will the path forward involve modifying a person's memory engram to allow them to recall a different experience of a disease or traumatic event, thereby transforming their psychological and physical states? This would revolutionize how providers treat chronic disease (including cancer and obesity).

Various pathways link NAFLD to obesity. "The emerging understanding of crosstalk between the liver and other organs complements and completes our knowledge of the role of hepatic immune regulation in liver disease development." (Zhang et al., 2022). "Obesity is not a consequence of a drug deficiency or a lack of willpower but a lack of knowledge of which nutrients are necessary and which concentrations that are required to control silent inflammation and therefore control appetite." (Sears & Ricordi, 2011). Other inflammatory mediators include epinephrine (Lelou et al., 2022), environmental toxins, pathogens (Yang Zhou, 2023), and *viruses, overburdening the liver and leading to dysfunction. Controlling ROS may control the cellular and molecular processes of liver fibrosis (Blas-García & Apostolova, 2023).

LiverTox® is an updated and unbiased website about causes and diagnosis of liver injury "attributable to prescription and nonprescription medications." An overburdened liver can cause acid reflux by decreasing bile production and increasing bacteria due to low hydrochloric acid (Llorente et al., 2017). Using acid reflux treatment as a long-time therapy stops the production of acid and allows enterococcus bacteria to thrive, leading to inflammation and worsening of NAFLD (Llorente et al., 2017).

Targeting inflammation can assist human livers in effectively performing vital metabolic and immunologic functions. Providers prescribing a low-fat or other specific diet can also consider detection and destruction of any present liver toxins and pathogens (prompting inflammation) to assist in optimal organ functioning. Hepatoprotection is enhanced by the professionally guided use of "certain foods, fruits, and plants." (Mega et al., 2021). Stress management and daily ingestion of whole food sources such as celery, onion, ginger, and turmeric boost the immune system (Singh et al., 2023). "In cancer, the apoptotic pathway is typically inhibited through a wide variety of means, including overexpression of antiapoptotic proteins and under-expression of proapoptotic proteins that cause resistance to chemotherapy." (Singh et al., 2023). Therefore, anticancer therapies derived from plants can activate the apoptotic pathway, leading to cancer cell destruction. (Singh et al., 2023). Have all potential determinants of inflammation and interventions been identified and addressed?

The immune system is compromised by pollution, radiation, and consumer products found to contain polyfluoroalkyl substances (PFAs). Hepatotoxicity has been found in humans as PFAs accumulate in the liver and other tissues (Costello et al., 2022), elevating ALT levels in people with NAFLD. Thus, the Environmental Protection Agency (EPA) continues to develop PFA remediation efforts. (EPA, 2022). How can providers take restorative actions without overburdening an already compromised liver? Consistent natural antioxidant and dietary B vitamin ingestion is required for biological processes, and vitamin B12 is needed for proper metabolism, myelination, and central nervous system function. (Singh et al., 2021). Vitamin B deficiencies can result in cognitive, cardiac, skin, and many other medical conditions (Singh et al., 2021). Some natural sources of B vitamins are found in salmon, leafy greens, bananas, meat, and dairy products. (Singh et al., 2021). However, can nutrients be properly absorbed in the presence of toxins in body organs?

Stigmas can exist for those diagnosed with certain diseases. Diagnostic labels like liver cirrhosis, obesity, mental illness, and cognitive impairment can prevent people from seeking professional assistance. Healthcare staff referring to patients by diagnosis, such as "the diabetic," or the "alcoholic" can suggest personal identification as a disease or invoke anger at its presence. These and all diagnoses imbuing a natural order of events placed within a perception of predictable outcomes, ensures its sustainability. Are individuals finding it challenging to achieve healing due to years or even decades of conditioning from society or the medical community? If so, they might struggle to break free from established consensus that has become deeply ingrained in their personal beliefs (Chapter 2).

Most patients are unaware of the crosstalk between the liver, pancreas, and other operatives involved in the complex diabetes chain of events. Antipsychotics or "APDs can cause serious glucometabolic side-effects including type 2 diabetes." (Chen et al., 2017). Overlapping physiologic contributions of the liver, pancreas, and adrenals add to glucose dysregulation. Sustained cortisol levels (consistently living in fight-or-flight) may add to adrenal fatigue and inflammation, modulating pancreatic beta-cell dysfunction and increasing the risk for type 2 diabetes. Some research articles link diabetes mellitus with *viral, bacterial, fungal, parasitic, and chemical agents. Endocrine disrupting chemicals (EDCs) can damage the "hypothalamus-pituitary, adrenal, and thyroid glands." (Egalini et al., 2022). "Type 1 diabetes mellitus… (T1DM) affecting β-cells may be initiated by environmental contaminants, such as per- and poly-fluoroalkyl substances (PFAS)." (Guarnotta et al., 2022) (Chapter 10).

Certain HMs*** (systemic toxicants) disrupting normal metabolic signaling pathways are associated with many chronic diseases, including diabetes, cancer, cardiovascular, neurodegenerative, and inflammatory diseases. (Haidar et al., 2023). Heavy metals are passed on in utero and can accumulate by eating foods from "contaminated soil, seafoods, and drinking water." (Haidar et al., 2023). Can this environmental factor contribute to or account for children being diagnosed with cancer or other chronic diseases?

**Many other constituents can compromise an immune system.** Within the stress system framework, Seyle's general adaptation syndrome is a "systematic stress response, while physical and mental disorders produced by prolonged stress are stress effects." (Lu et al., 2021). "Emotional, oxidative, mitochondrial, and metabolic stress" may trigger responses at the "molecular, cellular, and systemic levels." (Lu et al., 2021). Walter Cannon presented the theory of perceptions influencing emotions, triggering hormones that act upon the central nervous system and reticular activating system (Quick & Henderson, 2016). Occupational and environmental stressors can result in physical, psychological, and behavioral distress (Quick & Henderson, 2016). In this framework, "the **stress stimulus produces the effect, and the stressor, stress, and stress response are the cascade.**" (Quick & Henderson, 2016). Investigating and recognizing all constituents of disease assists in assessing a patient's potential need for multiple levels of support. **Providers may also consider offering psychological assistance (including but not limited to stress management) to enhance disease resistance and promote resilience.**

Type 1 diabetes (T1D) is described as an immunological response involving T-cell mediation of B-cell destruction. (Vandamme & Kinnunen, 2020). Multiple pathways, including Reactive oxygen species (ROS), play a role in beta cell destruction. "This is supported by the experimental data showing that the correction of ROS production and modulation of redox-related signaling and modifications by plant derived antioxidants (such as polyphenolic compounds) can stimulate pro-survival pathways in beta cells under diabetic condition." (Dinić et al., 2022). Monoclonal antibodies have been considered in newly diagnosed Type 1 diabetic patients. Mitigating metabolic factors modulating inflammation and oxidative stress may be found in probiotics, prebiotics, and synbiotics. (Iatcu et al., 2021). Enteroviruses, such as the Coxsackie B (CVB5) virus, are associated with an increased risk of T1D. (Isaacs et al., 2021). There is no T1D genetic connection in 85% of diagnosed TD1 children. (Isaacs et al., 2021). "We previously demonstrated that CVB5 infection leads to the significant dysregulation of multiple microRNAs that regulate the expression of a network of T1D risk genes in human pancreatic islets." (Isaacs et al., 2021). "Strategies targeting miRNAs and other endogenous factors or based on natural products such as bacterial compounds or plant extracts should be explored to fight against EVs infections and their effects on the host in order to prevent and/or treat T1D." (Nekoua et al., 2022). Then identifying, assessing, and targeting specific viral triggers must be expected to address diabetes risks, prevention, and in considering interventions.

Eradicating oxidative stress, fungi, bacteria, and viruses (Trinh, 2022) such as the enterovirus and Epstein-Barr Virus* (EBV) (Fevang et al., 2021) can help stop and correct inflammatory pathways that upset homeostasis. Hematopoietic stem cell transplantation and natural bioactive compounds found in fruits, vegetables, and plants may help treat EBV. (Wang et al., 2023). The pathogenesis of some chronic diseases is due to excess oxidants and chronic inflammation (Zhang et al., 2015). Oxidant and antioxidant imbalance facilitate molecular damage interrupting redox signaling (Jiang et al., 2021). Counteractants to oxidative stress include antioxidants and phytochemicals (Jiang et al., 2021). Medical providers might consider referring patients for nutritional counseling to bolster the immune system and support the body's natural detoxification processes.

Some practitioners and patients view medicine as operating within a one-size-fits-all approach. This does not allow for discrepancies arising from implementation of research data derived from different or imprecise populations (chapter 3). How can such errors be averted? Perhaps by specific lab testing for viruses and HMs, etc., evaluating an individual's nutritional state, and by defining each patient's personal explanation of disease. In an open atmosphere, patients can freely share their beliefs. Populations perceived pejoratively preclude clinicians from understanding individual perspectives. Medical anthropologist Arthur Kleinman, MD, proposed the explanatory model to clarify patient beliefs and expectations. (Kleinman & Benson, 2006). Acknowledging each patient's beliefs allows practitioners to learn about their mindset, coping mechanisms, engage with them on a more personal level, and understand what may resonate with them.

As anyone anywhere can believe another health system's dogma, disease pathology tenets and therapies, targeted questions reduce assumptions. Personal interpretations of origination of illness may include bad luck, divine influence, predestination, etc. These beliefs may be perceived as superstitions to a clinician but can be real to another. "Beliefs become a reality as this level of awareness becomes biochemistry." (Rao et al., 2009) (chapters 1 & 2). Cell biologist and scientific researcher Dr. Bruce Lipton, Ph.D., finds that the pattern of subconscious programming (habits) can be reprogrammed (brain rewiring). (Lipton, 2024). If one feels guilty for not doing everything to prevent their illness, can changing their perceptions modify their body chemistry? How does one believe the exacerbation, progression, and recurrence of their disease can be prevented? An individual's answers may provide insight into their interpretation of disease, though, judgment of their responses erodes trust. Can clinical medical anthropologists liaise bridging Western biomedicine and Eastern psychosocial elements of disease causation?

Practitioners following a holistic approach consider a variety of determinants by assessing multidimensional aspects of an individual then respond to physical or psychological manifestations accordingly. They examine all human embodiments and interactions in relation to physical injury, toxic and pathologic exposures, and emotional traumas as inflammatory influencers of illness and chronic disease. Cytokines, free radicals, UV-light (producing ROS), and X-Rays activate inflammation instigating chronic conditions. (Ciążyńska et al., 2021). Some "studies show inflammatory cytokines exert important effects with regard to various inflammatory diseases." (Kany et al., 2019).

There is a bidirectional immune-endocrine system interaction. (Klein, 2021). Lysosomal and mitochondrial dysfunction create the pathogenesis of neurodegenerative disorders like Alzheimer's and Parkinson's diseases. (Chen et al., 2022). "TRAP1" participates in lysosomal-mitochondrial crosstalk to maintain cellular homeostasis and could represent a potential therapeutic target for multiple disorders." (Chen et al., 2022). As well, practitioners can consider addressing circadian rhythm disturbances as outlined in chapter 4.

Bioactive compounds may activate encoded natural killer cells. "Subsequently, tremendous studies have shown that nutraceuticals derived from spices such as clove, coriander, garlic, ginger, onion, pepper, turmeric, etcetera., remarkably prevent and cure various chronic diseases by targeting inflammatory pathways." (Kunnumakkara et al., 2018). "It has been well established that the population who consume spices are less susceptible to the development of chronic diseases" (Kunnumakkara et al., 2018). Authors Kunnumakkara et al., (2018) also cite the anti-inflammatory properties of cilantro, parsley, and other fresh herbs to potentially ease and prevent chronic disease. Will private and government researchers and the NIH food as medicine study (chapter 5) conclusions reflect the findings of the researchers cited in this chapter and throughout this text to enhance naturally preventing and reversing chronic disease states?

"Vitamin C appears to be able to both prevent and treat respiratory and systemic infections by enhancing various immune cell functions." (Carr & Maggini, 2017). Consumed animal and dairy products treated with antibiotics and growth hormones Bovine somatotropin (bST) and estrogen have been considered suspects in increasing the propensity of breast tumors. Many dairy products carry labels advising that their cows were not treated with bST. "Current-use antibiotics and pesticides were undetectable in organic but prevalent in conventionally produced milk samples, with multiple samples exceeding federal limit." (Welsh et al., 2019).

Are vitamins supplying cell energy assisting in their biological cognizance? Some researchers have concluded that all organisms are sentient and work in collaboration. "Cognitive processing takes place in every single cell of our bodies, among which neuronal cells play a key part, but only a part." (Ciaunica et al., 2023). "Hence, one may say that we literally think with all the cells of our bodies, and not just our heads." (Ciaunica et al., 2023). "Recently, we have developed the cellular basis of consciousness (CBC) model, which proposes that all biological awareness, sentience, and consciousness are grounded in general cell biology." (Baluška et al., 2021). "Cells continuously rearrange their molecules according to their actual sensory experiences" and "bacteria use bioelectricity to establish memories and biocommunication." (Baluška et al., 2021). Can this model explain the existence of antibiotic-resistant bacteria? "Bacterial biofilm allows antibiotic resistance, though indole derivatives (phytochemicals) are a non-toxic approach to eliminate biofilm." (Odularu et al., 2022). Indole is naturally found in cruciferous vegetables (Esteve, 2020).

Although antibiotic therapy has saved lives, it can facilitate the pathogenesis of diseases. The bidirectional communication of gut microorganisms and the neuroendocrine system affects immune mediators (Chakrabarti et al., 2022). Frequent antibiotic administration in neonates and childhood corresponds with irritable bowel syndrome, obesity, and colorectal cancer (Patangia et al., 2022), neurodegenerative diseases (Chakrabarti et al., 2022) and type 2 diabetes (Ye et al.,

2022). Medical providers reconsidering habitual antibiotic usage in early life and adulthood may prevent chronic disease. Concerns about the short and long-term adverse health effects of antibiotic therapy incentivizes all medical facilities to establish or update an antibiotic stewardship program. Does adding probiotics really overcome existent antibiotic-resistant gut bacteria?

Chronic diseases are viewed as incurable as their root causes were never uncovered thus, remain unaddressed. My friend found it challenging to comprehend her ovarian cancer diagnosis (Preface & Introduction). She seemed to only fit the postmenopausal and age risk criteria, though at times said she felt lonely, sometimes experienced emotional flare-ups, and had confirmed having several ACEs. "In diseases where epigenetic mechanisms are changed, such as cancer, many genes show altered gene expression and inhibited genes become activated." (Curty et al., 2020). "Dysregulation of the sympathetic nervous system (SNS) and the hypothalamic-pituitary-adrenal (HPA) axis has been implicated in promoting angiogenesis, tumor cell proliferation and survival, alteration of the immune response and exacerbating inflammatory networks in the tumor microenvironment." (Colon-Echevarria et al., 2019). Could an emotional component have contributed to my friend's cancer diagnosis? Generally, emotions are not recognized as having a direct cancer cause-and-effect relationship, although data supports that chronic stress and stress hormones cause tumorigenesis and cancer development (Dai et al., 2020). And that stress induces various emotions that contribute to offsetting psychological and physical well-being.

The transcription and translation processes of emotions can affect gene expression. "The small genetic PAFs {population attributable factions} estimated here from studies of MZ {monozygotic} twins…cast further doubt on the notion that our inherited genomes are the primary causes of chronic diseases." (Rappaport, 2016). Nearly all recognized medical and emotional disorders have been linked to excessive inflammation and oxidative stress (Carter, 2021).

As Oxytocin exhibits mitochondria anti-inflammatory and antioxidative stress properties (Carter et al., 2022), **can giving, receiving, and feeling love make a difference through the consistent natural** release of it? Could early detection and mitigation of the EBV* have been one factor in preventing my friend's onset of cancer? **Over 95% of people globally carry the** EBV that is associated with epithelial cancers and lymphomas and "transforms human B cells into immortalized lymphoblastoid cell lines." (Münz, 2020). "T cell receptors against transforming latent EBV antigens, but also against early lytic viral gene products, might be protective for the control of EBV infection and associated oncogenesis." (Münz, 2020). Some researchers indicate that treatment with intravenous pharmacologic ascorbic acid administration may help eradicate a chronic EBV infection.

**Cited for its** limitations of explaining how psychosocial factors cause disease (Maydych, 2019), the **biopsychosocial model** may be a useful framework for comprehending mental illness. Practitioners viewing human beings holistically, can regard all dimensions that can affect the physical body. Bidirectional causal influences and emotions prompting inflammation and cellular responses (Maydych, 2019) may amplify the utility of this type of model. Thus, the variables of disease determinants may include sincerely investigating the causal roles of emotional, mental, socioeconomic, environmental, and spiritual states. Or determining what is prompting sentient cellular responses. The 3-P model "expands on *how* disease develops and is maintained," and considers all factors, "the predisposing, precipitating, and perpetuating factors instigating disease." (Wright et al., 2019). Acute and chronic psychosocial stressors including negative valence systems prompting inflammation are associated with the onset and recurrence of depression (Maydych, 2019) and other diseases. (Liu et al., 2017). "There is considerable evidence that psychological stress can activate the inflammatory response." (Maydych, 2019).

We can assess and address root causes if medicine considers all underlying mechanisms, including conscious and subconscious processes, that prompt physiological reactions (dysregulation and dysfunction). The disruption of homeostasis from chronic stress leads to various diseases like atherosclerosis, NAFLD, and depression (Liu et al., 2017). Chronic and acute stressors increase proinflammatory cytokines, promote inflammation, and tissue damage (Liu et al., 2017). Stress lowers immune system responses and increases risks for bacterial and viral infections.

Although there is no specific gene designated for mental illness (NIMH, 2020), a genetic component for mental illnesses and behavioral disorders is consistently implicated. Genes have been associated in the etiology of autism spectrum disorder (ASD), though several studies have proven causation resulting from epigenetic dysregulation (Wiśniowiecka-Kowalnik & Nowakowska, 2019). Studies show an epigenetic effect (heavy metal exposures) may form ROS and the development of ASD (Ding et al., 2023) and bipolar disorder. (Sampath et al., 2022).

Followers of non-reductionist views of Eastern medicine, such as Traditional Chinese Medicine and Ayurveda, may anticipate Allopathic, mind-body interventions, both, and neither. Anyone may be seeking mitigation of energetic Qi (chi) blockages of life force or Prana (life energy). Some believe an excess or deficiency of these energies vibrationally creates imbalances causing disease and disobeying the laws of the universe blocks chakras (energy centers) leaving one open to maladies. Perhaps when the reality of a person's truth defaults to sustained stress, opposition, and discordance, human cells respond with acute or chronic disease. Some individuals have discovered that focusing on love and personal peace can lead to a sense of wholeness. This personal evidence suggests that prioritizing emotional connections and inner tranquility can enhance one's overall well-being.

Western medicine (WM) agrees with Eastern medicines to the extent of replacing deficiencies and reducing whatever is in excess. And WM recognizes proximal causes and physical imbalances but not energetic ones. Energy has the potential to bridge Eastern and Western medicine. This connection could foster a more holistic approach to healthcare by integrating the strengths of both medical traditions. This convergence can broaden therapeutic options and promote a more comprehensive view of patient care, emphasizing the importance of balance among the mind, body, and spirit. Other medical systems and researchers within this chapter implicate the negative energetic imbalance of emotional states (below) contribute to disease states. However, there is no such definitive inventory to standardize recognizing and addressing these disease constituents at that level.

Can memory engram-encoded information allow a disease to resurface by reviving the original neural correlates? Does the inflammatory response serve as confirmation of this mechanism? Although engrams are reported to reside in brain structures, could attributions of negative emotions be stored in anatomical structures and visceral organs through cellular memory? Some government supported entities (chapter 5), heed researchers who have outlined that toxic emotions are stored and affect body organs and tissues. (Lee et al., 2017). Those government entities recognize that negative emotions from childhood traumatic events require intervention. Emotional components and psychosocial stress factors have been found to adversely contribute to physical, mental, and behavioral conditions.

Adverse childhood experiences** "(ACEs) from ages 0-17 include abuse, neglect, economic, family dysfunction," and other adverse situations as determinants of chronic disease, mental illness, and substance abuse. (CDC, 2021). These experiences impact psychological and physiological states affecting the immune, endocrine, and nervous systems. Some disease states related to ACEs include diabetes and depression. (Herzog & Schmahl, 2018). An ACE risk assessment can be considered as a routine screening process at every patient visit. Referrals for mental, emotional, and financial support, etcetera, may prevent complications in adulthood. A free noncopyrighted Behavioral Risk Factor Surveillance System survey can be accessed on the CDC website. Are all patients diagnosed with ACEs as children or adults receiving corresponding support?

PTSD can result from first-hand traumatic events or by proxy. Unresolved trauma can lead to anger, shame, guilt (Pai et al., 2017), depression, and possibly self-destructive actions. Can PTSD trigger somatic symptoms that are interpreted as unexplained? Providers and patients confronting suppressed psychological issues and emotions create a potential to mediate symptoms. Psychological interventions "are effective for managing PTSD symptoms and mental health comorbidities in people with complex-trauma histories." (Coventry et al., 2020).

If a psychopathological connection exists, investigating mind-body mechanisms and modalities is a consideration for identifying and reaching a source. Mind-body practices have shown efficacy in anxiety and depressive symptoms and symptomatic improvement in depression in PTSD patients. (Zhu et al., 2022). Evaluating work-related injury participants in an online imagery treatment program (replacing negative images with positive ones) was found to be an effective intervention. (Lee et al. 2018). Individual or group therapy, cognitive processing, and guided imagery may benefit people with PTSD. However, anyone, including military veterans feeling the stigma of a PTSD diagnosis may avoid seeking assistance. United States military veterans can access information and resources on this military website. Involving a supportive partner is helpful for those undergoing PTSD and depression therapy. Veterans considering private or couples therapy can also seek assistance through private enterprises (see end notes).

The complex etiology of depression includes emotional trauma, confirmed heavy metal*** exposure (Xia et al., 2022), and increased HPA axis activity from chronic stress. (Mikulska et al., 2021). Through the prism of nutritional psychiatry, low fruit and vegetable intake are associated with a higher risk of depression. (Li et al., 2017). Bipolar disorder is hypothesized to result from "the accumulation of EBV-infected autoreactive B cells with expected treatment by EBV-specific T-cell therapy." (Pender, 2020). Some people diagnosed with depression may have an inflammatory response from chronic and acute stress. Inflammation activating the sympathetic nervous (SNS) system sans parasympathetic counterbalance increases pro-inflammatory cytokines. (Pongratz & Straub, 2014). "Increased SNS activity, HPA activity, and the resultant chronic catabolic state leads to known comorbidities in chronic inflammatory disease, like cachexia, high blood pressure, insulin resistance, and increased cardiovascular mortality." (Pongratz & Straub, 2014) "While many factors play a role in the development of depression and fatigue, both have been associated with increased inflammatory activation of the immune system affecting both the periphery and the central nervous system (CNS)." (Lee & Giuliani, 2019). **What contributes to immune cells releasing inflammatory mediators?**

Human bodies can become vulnerable to and weakened by each emotional upset, stressor, and traumatic event Then mental, emotional, and spiritual factors can be seen as enhancing susceptibility or immunity. Researchers throughout this chapter and text have discovered that injury, toxins, pathogens, emotions, and stress can have synergistic inflammatory effects, which may lead to the development of disease. Other researchers (declining to share clinical trial findings) have found that these factors can contribute to idiopathic pain. This ongoing debate highlights the complexity of pain management and the need for a more integrated approach to treatment. Investigating the interplay between these variables could pave the way for more effective therapeutic strategies that address both the physical and psychological components of pain.

Acute and chronic stress is linked to emotional states inciting inflammation, metabolic, and other disorders. Then, emotions and infectious agents can work in tandem to effectuate or exacerbate disease states. "Epstein–Barr virus (EBV), parvovirus B19 (B19V), and human endogenous retroviruses (HERVs) are involved in SLE pathogenesis." (Quaglia et al., 2021). "We identified specific copies of *HERVK*, whose expression in the brain may be associated with ALS" (Moreno et al., 2024). The EBV infiltrates B lymphocyte cells. (Saha & Robertson, 2019). EBV effectuates malignancies, rheumatoid arthritis, and diseases like MS and lupus. (Fugl & Andersen, 2019) (Trier et al., 2018). MS is not proven to originate in the CNS or by autoimmune mechanisms. (Jung et al., 2019). "These results cannot be explained by any known risk factor for MS and demonstrate that EBV is the leading cause of MS." (He et al., 2022). However, not all EBV carriers exhibit symptoms or are diagnosed with a disease. So, what is the etiology for the EBV to activate and create disease?

Heavy metals, organic solvents, and chemical exposure can contribute to MS onset and disease progression. (Hachim et al., 2019). "In general, EBV can enter the body via direct infection or indirectly via B-cell invasion, enter the CNS by regulating the function of B- or T-lymphocytes, and cause neuroinflammation and immune disorders, finally leading to the development of nervous system diseases." (Zhang et al., 2022). The latent EBV (can stimulate ROS) and is reactivated by infections including COVID-19, and psychological stressors. (Sausen et al., 2021).

Understanding pathological constituents of disease may advance if researchers can identify the multiple strains and mutations of EBV and bacteria some researchers find catalyze inflammatory bowel and other common diseases. Some viruses, including live enteroviruses and HHV-6 have been found in the thyroid gland (Weider et al., 2022). Are these viruses an agent prompting thyroid diseases, Ehlers-Danlos Syndrome, immune-mediated and other diseases, disorders, or unexplained symptoms? Proinflammatory interleukins incite flu-like symptoms in chronic fatigue syndrome (CFS). (Yang et al., 2019). Patients with CFS have increased oxidative stress. "Oxidative stress, a status of excessive ROS generation exceeding the capacity of antioxidant defense, is known to be involved in a wide range of pathophysiological processes, such as inflammation, vascular disorder, cancer, aging, and chronic fatigue." (Lee et al., 2018). This can lead to molecular and cellular damage as free radicals result in less energy and damage mitochondria. Researchers previously cited, have reviewed how antioxidants interrupt the transmission of free radicals and reduce inflammation.

Albert Einstein said, "We cannot solve our problems with the same thinking we used when we created them." This statement reinforces that changing our thoughts can produce different results, though it insinuates that conditions are self-generated. Disease sufferers are not to blame, as not all medical systems recognize the full effect that psychological factors influencing emotions and exogenous determinants have on the physical layer. Including that anything (a positive or negative effect) is possible if one believes. Not investigating the extent of beliefs creating personal truth (chapter 2), the spiritual dimension, and the extent that vibrations and frequencies (Chapter 8) have on disease states may leave chronic disease entities unaddressed. Einstein believed in the physics of vibrations as chemical and electrical charges change cells. "Compelling evidence is presented, showing that biological patterns are strongly embedded in the vibrational nature of the physical energies that permeate the entire universe." (Tassinari et al., 2022). "We hope that these efforts will boost the chance among the scientific community of using mechanical vibrations, bioelectricity, and electromagnetic radiation (including light) to develop innovative approaches in the control of epigenetics, tissue morphogenesis, and regeneration, even paving the way for offering additional tools in the handling of oncogenesis and metastatic spreading." (Tassinari et al., 2022).

When two systems exchange energy, they also exchange information. This relationship is important in fields like thermodynamics and information theory, where the flow of energy often corresponds with the flow of information. If energy and matter are interchangeable (Einstein's equation

$E=mc^2$), then can disease imbalances be resolved within this framework? Understanding how energy fluctuations (vibrations and frequencies) can influence matter at the cellular level, paves the way for the development of innovative therapies that restore balance and promote healing.

Some government supported entities (chapter 5), believe the soul receives messages from emotional, mental, or spiritual imbalances within the body where human burdens settle. That is, the body communicates information through the type of symptoms the body part needs to release by arising to the surface for healing. Research into the advantages of a framework including spiritual aspects influencing disease, may advance current medical models by recognizing and addressing humans as multidimensional beings.

Belief or doubt in divinity is a personal choice therefore, the following can sound natural to those living in a perception of spirituality and unnatural to those who don't. The spiritual onset of sickness is attributed to spiritual distress including a disconnect from others, absence of inner peace (Klimasiński et al., 2022), purpose, and separateness from a spiritual source. Depression and anxiety have increased with poor spiritual perceptions (Mendes et al., 2023). "As all therapy is psychotherapy, so all illness is mental illness." Judgment is a decision, made again and again, against creation and its Creator. It is a decision to perceive the universe as you would have created it. It is a decision that truth can lie and must be lies. What, then, can illness be except an expression of sorrow and of guilt?" (ACIM, P-2.IV.1:1-7).

A common perception is that certain diseases are inevitable, expected, or age-related. Although amyloid plaques research began in the 1980s, it is just now being considered in Alzheimer's Disease (AD). HMs*** aggravate viruses and can precipitate disease and AD. Oxidative stress is "induced by free radical formation." (Jaishankar et al., 2014), signaling the "pathogenesis of multiple human diseases." (Jan et al., 2015). Metals are found in some pharmaceuticals and foods and are passed on in utero. Toxic metals contribute to chronic illness by disrupting cellular events. (Balali-Mood et al., 2021), distort energy, communication, and block natural resonance. Can the buildup of toxic metals contribute to more prevalent diseases, such as depression, skin conditions, and certain cancers?

The aging population may exhibit general symptoms of chronic accumulation of HMs, (gastrointestinal disturbances, dysrhythmias, paresthesia, etc.). Metals like mercury in dental amalgams, fish, some meds, aluminum, copper, and stainless-steel products contribute to toxicity. Environmental metal exposure poses an opportunity for prion diseases due to the binding of prion proteins. (Toni et al., 2017). Will it become standard for patients to be prescreened for HMs to prevent cognitive decline? And for those with known or suspected exposure to HMs and accompanying symptoms to be assessed for toxic HM levels to prevent worsening?

As emphasis is placed on preparing for the onslaught of the aging population, awareness of causes in cognitive decline is required for prevention and intervention. Neurotoxicants include excessive arsenic (Thakur et al., 2021) lead and cadmium that associate with attention deficit hyperactivity disorder (ADHD). (Lee et al., 2018). The decreased antioxidant glutathione level increases oxidative stress and is associated with diabetes, neurodegenerative diseases, cancer, and age-related diseases (Minich & Brown, 2019). Glutathione is found in citrus fruits, green tea, avocados, and curcumin and may help in reducing toxic HMs (Minich & Brown). Lead mitigation includes replacing lead pipes and paint, removing shoes indoors, and handwashing (Lee et al., 2018).

Concerns about the aluminum byproduct fluoride added to public water systems exist. Fluoride is also found in the air and many organic and inorganic products that humans encounter or use. Fluoride belts are found in many countries, and most countries in Europe don't use water fluoridation because of the health risks. While some tout cavity protection, others find ethical concerns in fluoridation, as one cannot consent to something some researchers classify as a medication and harmful. Fluoride-free product data and fluoride-removing water filters can be evaluated in the end notes. Chlorine added for disinfection to public drinking water has also come under scrutiny. Chlorine and organic humic interactions in water give rise to carcinogenic and mutagenic substances (Kopler et al., 2022). Certain filters designed for chloramine removal include reverse osmosis and catalytic carbon filters. Some researchers propose boiling water, UV radiation, and activated carbon adsorption for removing organic compounds and pathogens. Non-carbon nanomaterials as sorbents help remove heavy metals from wastewater (Baby et al., 2022).

Persistent organic pollutants (pesticides and industrial chemicals) have been implicated as endocrine disruptors. Pesticides accumulating in adipose tissue disrupt endocrine functioning (Barrett, 2013) contributing to type 2 diabetes (Chapter 10). The FDA regulates pesticides in the U.S. and communicates with other countries. However, some countries may still be using banned pesticides posing a risk to produce, ecosystems, and all life (Beyond Pesticides, 2020). Although DDT is banned in the U.S. it is still used in some countries. The wind carrying pesticides over long distances, are detected in the soil of other countries (Beyond Pesticides, 2020). Multiple pesticides have been found in U.S. streams and rivers (U.S. Geological Survey, 2017, 2020). Some use a water test kit or obtain water samples for testing to check for contaminants.

This chapter has cited a fraction of clear and compelling research article consensus for translational debate and implementation science (Gunn et al., 2022). Scoping reviews can improve synthesizing information (Munn et al., 2018). When the medical community invests in researching root causes of diseases instead of symptom management (perceived as palliative care), medical consumers and providers can realize the mission of the medical profession.

Impeccable research practices and funding for root causes of chronic disease can establish disease pathology for accurate and precise prevention and healing measures. Each clinician perceiving beyond limitations can review diverse research papers to determine if findings can benefit themselves and humanity. Focusing on the underlying mechanisms of disease prevents reoccurrence, worsening, and development of chronic conditions. Research findings from all chapters can spur new perspectives of disease prevention, which is the essence of medical practice.

Identifying and addressing the underlying causes of chronic disease guides precise prevention measures. As old age is not a diagnosis, it is not necessarily the leading factor in chronic medical conditions or death. Therefore, it is necessary to examine the factors contributing to what people may erroneously be referring to as inevitable and unavoidable age-related diseases.

# Chapter 7

## Prevention: The Core of Clinical Practice

**"Disease can rarely be eliminated through early diagnosis
or good treatment, but prevention can eliminate disease."
~ Dennis Burkitt**

**"The aim of medicine is to prevent disease and prolong life, the
ideal of medicine is to eliminate the need of a physician."
~ William James Mayo**

**"You don't stop laughing when you grow old, you grow old
when you stop laughing." ~ George Bernard Shaw**

**"Watch your thoughts, they become your words; watch your
words, they become your actions; watch your actions, they
become your habits; watch your habits, they become your
character; watch your character, it becomes your destiny."
~ Lao Tzu**

Each day, one hundred-seven-year-old home vintner Antonio Docampo Garcia enjoyed consuming a bottle of red wine with each meal. At 124, Lola Francisca Susano's lifestyle included a plant-based diet devoid of alcohol. Did Thelma Sutcliffe's primordial prevention efforts of leading a stress-free life help her reach 115? If people of various lifestyles and healthcare systems lived beyond centenarian-hood, then is it possible for anyone? Was there a way these supercentenarians could have avoided collective perceptions of archetypal aging and demise? Did these elders eventually expect and accept the collective view of inevitable cognitive or physical decline? Is this perspective guiding current seniors and clinicians?

Equating life advancement with certain conditions precludes consideration of the cumulative effects of oxidative stress, DNA damage (Berben et al., 2021), and inherited or current exposure to toxic substances* (chapter 6). Was there early recognition of and attention to cellular mechanisms to prevent physical and mental decline? A person's age does not cause illness or demise. Seniors and their healthcare providers may not understand the full impact of toxins, pathogens, *heavy metals, and adverse childhood experiences (ACEs) on gene expression and disease (chapter 6). Chemicals released from toxins or emotions can affect sentient cells (Introduction, chapter 6), thus, health. The commitment of scientific research to consider the multifactorial qualifiers of disease will ultimately lead to creating prevention efforts.

Some physical and mental illnesses once explained by genetics are now viewed through the lens of epigenetics (environmental factors influencing gene expression). Once deemed impossible, completion of the human genome sequence was accomplished in 2022. Identification of genome variances may potentially lead to personalized health guidance. (NIH, 2022). So, what overarching means exist now to prevent the collectively proclaimed inevitable aging process and predictive "age-related" illnesses? Primary prevention methods, including attention to nutrition and oral health, can reduce and modify risks to prevent disease in the susceptible. Identifying all potential disease triggers (chapter 6) is the cornerstone of disease prevention. By understanding triggers and the **accurate determinants of biological age**, medical providers and patients can form personalized plans to avoid chronic disease.

**The number of years one has lived (chronological age) can vary from the health and function of a person's cells (biological age)**. As chronological age is not a cause of disease or death and chronic conditions are seen in the young, another metric has emerged (Wu et al., 2021). Focus has shifted to recognizing one's biological age based on epigenetic aging signals (Wu et al., 2021). DNA methylation is associated with aging and chronological age differs from DNA methylation age (Bin-Jumah et al., 2022).

Secondary prevention measures (identifying the biomarkers of inflammation) may predict conditions and offer a targeted response. **Diets high in calories and low in nutrients and neutraceuticals can catalyze disease and aging prematurely** (Poeggeler et al., 2023). Other epigenetic variables influencing metabolic regulatory pathways and immune functioning include dietary and supplemental choices, physical activity, and psychological factors. Through fMRI validation, "Mindfulness has shown an improved anti-inflammatory response and healthy aging by appropriate telomerase regulation." (Jamil et al., 2023).

The regulatory mechanism of dietary strategies can target cancer epigenetic pathways (Montgomery & Srinivasan, 2019) and affect aging. Epigenetic changes in ncRNA methylation (Bure et al., 2022) seen in cancer, aging, and other diseases can be mediated through caloric control while meeting nutrient requirements. (Fang et al., 2021). Choosing any degree of caloric restriction or fasting is best done under the supervision of your personal qualified licensed healthcare provider. Do practitioners believe it is too late for preventative teaching because a person is considered aged or may already have one or more chronic conditions?

Chronic medical conditions can be prevented and diminished through natural approaches. The vitamins and flavonoids in cruciferous vegetables and fruits may prevent chronic diseases including neurological and some cancers. (Connolly et al., 2021). The chemical properties of epigenetic dieting highlights cruciferous vegetables (medicinal bioactive metabolites) in preventing and treating colorectal cancer. (Ağagündüz et al., 2022).

Many autobiographies detail how the writer survived terminal cancer by changing certain daily practices. The oxidative effects of plant extracts and phenolic compounds have antiaging, anti-inflammatory, and chemoprotective properties. (Rahman et al., 2021). There is a growing interest in learning about nutrition for boosting immunity to maintain homeostasis. Therefore, from 2020-2030, the NIH is studying nutritional science and food as medicine (Chapter 5). Can the gap between phytochemical reactions of antioxidants and emotional turmoil at the time of cellular organ rejuvenation create an opportunity for disease? Chronic disease pathogenesis instigated by oxidative stress and free radicals, may be mitigated by the body's natural and nutritional defenses. (Sharifi-Rad et al., 2020).

Dysbiosis leading to gut inflammation may contribute to neuroinflammation and neurogenerative diseases. The bidirectional influence between the brain and gut may prompt gut microbiome interactions that are associated with the development and progression of Alzheimer's Disease, depression, and multiple sclerosis. (Mohajeri, 2019). The natural polyphenols in berries oxidative can mitigate oxidative stress and inflammation (Golovinskaia & Wang, 2021) and act on transcription factors. (Rahman et al., 2021). The bioactive compounds in berries other fruits and vegetables hold antiviral, antifungal, and antiparasitic properties and may lower risks for diseases including cancer and diabetes. (Rahman et al., 2021). The antiviral and immune protective mechanisms are found in spices, root vegetables, spirulina, and mushrooms. (Rahman et al., 2021). Contact your healthcare provider(s) to diagnose a possible vitamin deficiency and provide guidance on potential supplements and food sources for any diagnosed condition or prevention purposes.

Dual identity as a medical professional and patient does not imply acumen for non-prescribed nutritional substitutes or other therapies. Clinicians may be reluctant to ask their healthcare provider or pharmacist about potential interactions with prescribed and over-the-counter medications or supplements. Within their framework, the FDA does not approve supplements before they are marketed but can enforce their laws if they find any misbranded or adulterated dietary supplement after marketing. (FDA, 2022). Supplements can be removed if audits find them unsafe, misleading or false. (FDA, 2022). Anyone can report safety concerns of dietary supplements, human biologics, and animal food and drugs on the FDA reporting site.

Some providers doubt that vitamin or mineral supplementation reduces disease risks or cognitive decline. And that a healthy diet should provide all needed nutrients. However, many people use them as a prevention measure anyway. Though, interpretations of a nutritious diet can vary and adherence to a prescribed diet can be difficult for persons considered a high-risk for vitamin deficiencies. A vitamin D deficiency is linked to chronic diseases such as "bone metabolic disorders, tumors, cardiovascular diseases, and diabetes." (Wang et al., 2017). Oxidative damage can disrupt healthy aging (shorten telomeres) due to lower amounts of vitamins C, E, zinc, and selenium. (Kaźmierczak-Barańska et al., 2020). It is not enough to eat well if nutrients cannot be properly absorbed in the presence of toxins (Chapter 6).

Orthomolecular medicine that centers on individual biochemistry to correct molecular imbalances and prevent chronic disease is often ignored. Generally, orthomolecular practitioners, Naturopaths, or a Doctor of Osteopathy (DO) specialize in verifying a need for high dosage of intravenous vitamin C to correct imbalances.

A newer strategy may provide a theoretical reference for preventing and treating obesity and type 2 diabetes. This involves employing methods to burn fat by browning excess white fat to "protect against obesity and obesity-related metabolic disease." (Liu et al., 2023). "Berberine has been reported to exhibit anti-diabetic activity and to improve disordered lipid metabolism" (Zhu et al., 2018). As well, resveratrol may protect against diabetes. (Su et al., 2022).

Resveratrol modulates molecular signaling pathways to exert cardioprotective effects, including "antioxidative stress, anti-inflammatory, antiapoptotic, and pro-autophagic." (Song et al., 2020). Degradation mechanisms leading to cartilage damage and osteoarthritis development are further affected by non-coding RNA (ncRNA) expression directing disease progression. (Gu et al., 2022). Since epigenetic changes can be modulated, targeting specific signaling pathways may deactivate the collaborative ncRNA effects. That is, in mediating the effects of inflammation to reduce cartilage degeneration and regulate IL-6 expression it mediates other signaling cascades. (Ghafouri-Fard et al., 2021).

Attention to encouraging the biological processes such as apoptosis (normal programmed cell death), helps restore homeostasis. (Zhang, et al., 2022). Dysfunction of essential cell removal catalyzes viral and bacterial diseases, and degenerative and neurogenerative diseases. (Xu et al., 2019). Targeting the energy of impaired cellular and molecular mechanisms of aging includes attention to oxidative stress (Buoso et al., 2022) helps prevent inflammatory responses. "Tumor necrosis factor receptor-associated protein 1 (TRAP1) to prevent aging is able to prevent oxidative stress-induced cell death." (Faienza, et al., 2020). Trap 1 modulation may mediate cellular reactive oxygen species (free radicals) contributing to aging and possibly regulate its pathophysiology. (Faienza, et al., 2020). Through apoptotic pathways, nontoxic anticarcinogenic (curcumin and other plant derivatives) may be considered for "more universal cancer therapy." (Pfeffer & Singh, 2018). Some researchers say that late-stage cell reversal can be achieved through washing away apoptotic stimuli.

Previous researchers implicate the underlying mechanisms (energy) prompting the physiological reactions, causing dysregulation and dysfunction are emotional. What is the mindset (conscious or mindless?) while ingesting food, prescribed medications and therapies, and supplements? Some hold intentions of what is being consumed to empower the chemical to exert the desired effect. In the presence of personal peace (chapter 10), they can be seen as being allowed to effectively perform their functions. One can choose to believe in the same, comfortable, and routine or become curious about what biomedical scientists and lifestyle clinic researchers are finding and the interventions that have been working for people. Can we learn anything from our ancient ancestors?

Millions worldwide accept the documentation of hundreds of years old human beings as described in sacred texts. Others view supercentenarian individuals and groups in religious or ancient cultures as resembling apocryphal lore. Then, collective thinking can translate to a personal theory of impossibility. Did these ageless beings imagine beyond the limits of human understanding and choose the beliefs that created their reality? Were the supercentenarians described in Holy Writs centered on defying aging by connecting to and maintaining the highest Divine universal vibration and frequency (Chapter 8)? Did their spiritual relationship and beliefs allow regeneration and rejuvenation and the impetus to forestalling aging, decay, and an early death? Were the ancients able to maintain their immune systems by perceiving food as medicinal? **Did they consistently use sound and music (vibrational therapy and other natural and transcendental energies) for healing and health maintenance? And use humor and laughter increasing endorphins consistently making them feel good (influencing sentient cells)? Was the aging process delayed through nonjudgment, inner peace (chapter 10), and their connection to pure love? Did disease yield to a natural transcendent state? Had aging slowed as people consistently mindful (always living in the present)?**

As people witnessed others achieving supercentenarian status, was longevity then accepted as the standard? Were the ancients in harmony with their bodies because they addressed all bodily dimensions and everything else affecting epigenetics before a disease could actualize? Is it definite that among the uncontacted peoples and tribes in the world, two-hundred-year-old people have never existed or are not currently living? "Absence of evidence does not mean evidence of absence." (Dr. Carl Sagan). **Did the elders believe connecting with and maintaining divine frequencies could change the seemingly stochastic nature of the laws operating within the universe?** Had the ancients considered the energy of natural dietary factors in achieving and maintaining immune protection and emotional health (Chapter 6)? And did they believe in the power of always being conscious to prevent personal or work-related accidents and injuries (Chapter 8)? The Consciousness Research Interest Group offers scientific seminars on the science of consciousness (NIH, 2023).

Consideration of multidimensional assessments including consciousness-based **ones into healthcare practice represents a** transformative approach to patient care. Patients articulating their experiences and feelings more effectively, lead providers to a deeper understanding of their health concerns. By prioritizing the mental and emotional aspects of physical health, healthcare providers can create a more personalized therapeutic treatment framework.

Preventing illness also prevents cost burdens of disease manifestation and their potential complications. Prevention of mental illness in adulthood may be precluded by early detection and intervention of adverse childhood experiences (ACEs) in childhood. (Thomas et al., 2016). Chronic diseases can be prevented by recognizing and addressing ACEs (emotional components that can affect the physical) and other suspected disease catalysts (Chapter 6). Attention to multidimensional factors may prevent reoccurrence of previous conditions.

Global medical communities are projecting a marked increase in the aging population. Globally, the number of seniors may reach over 1.5 billion by 2050. (The Population Division of the United Nations, 2019). It is predicted that the senior growth rate in the U.S. will nearly double from 2012 to 83.7 million by 2050. (United States Census Bureau, 2021). Worldwide, healthcare sectors are concerned about the physical and cognitive challenges of an aging population. Instead of seeing a global burden, researchers and healthcare professionals can be in the energy of the answers by being curious, open, and asking the most salient questions without preconceived answers. Review of disparate open and transparent research can guide medicine toward a framework in approaching prevention and "age-related" conditions (Chapter 6). This focus may help customize the desired ends of education, prevention, and delivering real solutions to medical consumers. As society cannot continue to do the same things expecting different results. (Albert Einstein), other protective measures must be expediently determined to increase life expectancy and quality.

Prevention imbues experiencing and maintaining an unencumbered existence. Continual protection relies upon the body's innate and adaptive immunity to maintain homeostasis. Perspectives of the aged populations' cognitive and immune functioning, deemed to diminish over time, makes diagnosing and treating these conditions routine. Researchers' findings of disease pathology (chapter 6) can guide apparent prevention recommendations for many "age-related" diseases. Preventing and intercepting the cumulative burdens of harmful substances (HMs, toxins, pathogens) (chapter 6) contributing to cognitive, degenerative, neurodegenerative diseases and psychosocial dimensions prevents suffering. Equally crucial to the corporeal, but less recognized, is maintaining emotional equilibrium (stress prevention) in averting disease states.

Multitudes consider the power of love to be a protective and healing mechanism. Many centenarians regard laughter, purpose, and spiritual and social connections as integral parts of the human defense apparatus. When psychological and numinous needs are met, in a balanced state, biological processes including correct cell regeneration and rejuvenation can commence. Precise cell division can then be influenced by a person's emotions and cognizance. What is the emotional level, mood, and nutritional state of the individual during sentient cell regeneration?

Many have perceived others as engaging in lifestyles considered to be a threat to their health. Forcing someone to break a habit and possible pleasure associated with these behaviors fosters resistance. Risk perceptions can be assessed for improved decision-making and motivational change. Those at risk and indifferent about potential negative outcomes may not be readily receptive to quitting tobacco products or other substances. Many find antismoking ads effective, though some smokers may believe quitting is not worth risking weight gain. This may be prevented by creating a healthy menu with one's healthcare provider, registered dietician, or nutritionist before selecting a quit date.

Though triggers, and cravings can arise. Neuroscience may help in modulating conditioned habits. Real-time fMRI neurofeedback, "Trains subjects to adjust brain neural activity autonomously to improve cognition or cure diseases." (Li et al., 2022). This amygdala-based training improved the sleep of patients with chronic insomnia and can improve symptoms of depression, anxiety, schizophrenia and other disease. (Li et al., 2022).

Reviewing patient understanding of medications upon discharge from inpatient or outpatient services can prevent improper usage. Some people have reported taking a prescribed medication every six hours when it was ordered Q6H PRN (every six hours as needed). As well, some patients perceived an antibiotic ordered every 12 hours could be taken twice any time within 24 hours. Pharmacists can continue to commit to this type of specific teaching to prevent adverse effects. The Agency for Healthcare Research and Quality's (AHRQ) re-engineered discharge toolkit (RED) may reduce these types of patient misperceptions to prevent medication errors. (AHRQ, 2020).

Clinicians involved in community prevention efforts can be effective in changes that prevent or reduce environmentally related and other diseases. Community awareness of local environmental issues affecting health may inspire corrective actions. Education of the Childhood Lead Poisoning Prevention Program and National Heart Disease and Stroke Prevention Program (CDC), toxic chemical exposures (indoor and outdoor contaminants, (chapter 10) may prevent cellular damage or death. As well, public health teaching can consider including education about the significance of heavy metals and common pathogens on health (Chapter 6). Then there can be awareness of targeted prevention and correction of specific stimuli triggering certain responses.

Previous chapters observed how professionals lived in crisis and traumatic stress during the 2020 global pandemic. This chapter sees that it called attention to prevention measures (covering a cough, hand hygiene, etc.) and the care of chronic conditions to reduce the chance of contracting the coronavirus. Many healthcare professionals encountered undue stress and psychological trauma, adding to contemporaneous workforce demands. Some medical workers experienced post-traumatic stress arising from contracting the coronavirus and witnessing large-scale human suffering. As coronavirus admissions grew, many professional workers felt overwhelmed by safety and potential ethical considerations. In 2020 and 2021, a significant fraction of the world population ventured outside their healthcare system as they consulted the Internet about how to heal and for mental health assistance. While local, state, and federal agencies responded to support clinicians, reactive medicine cannot sustain medical workers or patients in a wide-scale emergency. It is compulsory that the medical community develop proactive steps to comprehensively address and prevent this scenario before it can reoccur.

A silent online movement endures while searchers await government-sponsored clinical trial conclusions of potential naturopathic concepts. Will the integration of this prospective translational research complement clinician-preferred website information-gathering for real change? Or will it change the way health care providers view patients (as a whole, rather than just a diseased body part)? Disorders in one part of the body can affect the interrelationships and functions of other parts or the entire system. Chapter 6 detailed the power of personal belief in the expression of disease and healing. Looking beyond, the input of clinicians reviewing disparate research articles will mark the difference between indifference and effective action. Then, healthcare systems will be compelled to ascertain every facet of disease formulation for precise interventions.

Medical systems acting within an objective mindset, can perceive beyond the confines of collective limiting thought. They can consider a plethora of research papers in all chapters and other governments that attribute mental, emotional, spiritual, environmental, and social contributions for correct disease prevention and therapy. Can healthcare providers allow themselves to perceive beyond limitations to be part of a new collective reality? If so, this culture of proactive-thinking, forward-thinking, and divergent-thinking generates the ability of new and effective solutions.

The next chapter explores the interconnectedness of all human factors in healing as medical and allied health schools only partially address it. Professional congruency of diverse open and transparent systematic data in curriculum helps students define client priorities, healing perceptions, and the translational research capacity to address them. Chapter 8 will explore how insights from biomedical research can be utilized to enhance our understanding of natural influence. It strives to establish a connection between scientific discoveries and their practical implementation in the medical field.

# Chapter 8

## Healing Power

**"The most common way people give up their power is by thinking they don't have any."** ~ Alice Walker

**"All matter originates and exists only by virtue of a force which brings the particle of an atom to vibration and holds this most minute solar system of the atom together. We must assume behind this force the existence of a conscious and intelligent mind. This mind is the matrix of all matter."** ~ Max Planck

**"There is obviously only one alternative, namely the unification of minds or consciousnesses. Their multiplicity is only apparent, in truth there is only one mind."** ~ Erwin Schrödinger

Having rejected conventional treatment, she was on her own. In her book, Miracles from the Light (Publish America, 2007), Rosemary recounts her self-healing from laboratory-verified and physician-confirmed uterine cancer. Many people with incurable cancers have reported spontaneous cures, either after a near-death experience (NDE) or without one (non-NDE). The reports from both groups reveal striking similarities that warrant further investigation to achieve a more comprehensive understanding of the subject. By analyzing these findings, researchers may identify underlying patterns that could provide insights, solutions, and guidance for future studies.

Some people recount reversing terminal and chronic medical conditions through their spiritual connection, diet, prayer, or a combination of natural practices and supernatural experiences. The medical community often dismisses the explanations provided by NDE survivors, despite physician documentation and clear evidence of their spontaneous remissions. A person who instantly heals from a terminal disease or in the absence of conventional medical intervention is generally considered an anomaly, an aberration, or an outlier. Healthcare providers remain dubious about spontaneous healings, as precise mechanisms have not been substantiated by scientific evidence, notwithstanding the challenges linked to research studies (chapter 3).

"Spontaneous healing involves an intentional effect of a cause that transcends the logical mind." (Dispenza, 2022). This understanding among researchers has not motivated research funders to prioritize investigations into instantaneous healing. One factor may be that the medical definition of spontaneous remission does not imply a permanent state of being. Though, neither do some of the current conventional therapeutic approaches for chronic disease. However, many NDE survivors report they continue to live in the state of cure. When researching unexplained human experiences, curiosity devoid of preconceived expectations may connect anecdotal accounts, clinical insights, and professional prognostics. The ambiguity of spontaneous remissions either by an NDE or without an NDE, attributed to various theories, lead providers to dismiss the cured person and their experience. While not everyone has had the same exact experience, there are some similarities between the spontaneously healed. Many autobiographies in both groups describe feeling the energy of a pure unwavering love, healing light, and seeing themselves as whole. While these essences sound overly simplistic to reverse a complex disease process, they can inspire further investigation into these phenomena, the extent of the mind-body connection, and the broader implications of vibrations and frequencies in catalyzing healing (wholeness).

While medicine attempts to use the same standard therapies for healing, intentional mechanisms required for transmutation are disregarded. Replicated intention experiments involving non-local healing found that patients diagnosed with the acquired human immunodeficiency virus and cardiac patients in the prayer group healed faster than those treated with just conventional medicine (Dossey, 2020). Consciousness-based medicine also operates when a client's consciousness is used to affect their body chemistry. (Ventegodt et al., 2004).

Recognizing how beliefs can affect biochemistry. (Rao et al., 2009) (chapters 1 & 2) may help close the gap between general health care and whole-health care. The powerful desire to be well has driven many people to venture outside of their healthcare system. Some individuals perceiving a broader spectrum of options are conducting their own investigations, which sometimes include researching quantum healing. They point to lifestyle centers have reversed some chronic conditions, divergent biomedical research findings, and documentation of others having experienced instant healing. These latter patient action directly challenges the current scientific experimentation process. Then, how can different healing approaches achieving the same outcome work towards standardizing care?

When attempting to understand NDEs or anything unexplainable, arbitrary explanations and limiting beliefs create gaps. It can be perceived as challenging to review all scientific literature and form conceptual and theoretical frameworks to complement the collective knowledge of spontaneous recovery. And within the current concept of evidence, science must confirm how these healing instances are possible for everyone. Has the current medical model advanced to consistently claim this success? If not, then how can medicine offer a more realiable healing model? Objectivity and asking the best questions without preconceived answers paves the way to discovering the truth or drill down (chapter 5).

This chapter highlights an inventory of free will expressed throughout the world. Will biases lead to an immediate rejection of diverse information, or as physicians and the spontaneously healed have documented the perceived impossible, how can it not be possible? Perceiving beyond limitations requires transcending conventional thinking. However, logical thinking leads to determining whether something is likely, possible, or probable. When probability is defined by the odds (Preface), the prospect of healing is limited by chance. However, many believe that nothing is random while acting under the basic laws of physics, natural laws, and universal laws. Then, everything that occurs is governed by underlying principles and forces, implying that events are interconnected and predictable within the framework of these laws. Then, one may conclude that events are not random unless they choose to interpret them as such.

Viewing things from a broader perspective (in objectivity, free from emotions, and judgments) allows for the recognition of various potentials. In medicine, can everyone be expected to conform to specific models of prediction? Or, considering that beliefs shape reality (chapter 2), can perceiving beyond limiting beliefs alter individual experiences? When using research as a reference, were clinical trial participants wholly representative of the target population and was the study bias-free? If experience consistently guides the future, how can anything ever be different for another if the same assumptions always predict outcomes?

"We do not learn from experience...we learn from reflecting on experience." (John Dewey).

People's perspectives on life may help them transcend limitations. Decades ago, a friend echoed Eleanor Roosevelt when she stated, "Life is what you make it," while not ruling out the possibility of the life experience as being a test or a game. Then, one can strategize to overcome life's issues within this clinical trial of human actions and reactions. My friend was unaware of Albert Einstein's statement that, "Life is just like a game; first, you have to learn the rules of the game and then play it better than anyone else." Within this construct, everyone raised within this collective consciousness must balance personal experiences translating to their (repetitive subconscious thoughts) affecting emotions and reality. Perceiving life as a game is not about competitiveness but about each person becoming the best version of themselves.

"The mind is everything; what you think, you become." (Gautama Buddha). Many researchers consider the human psyche to be a multidimensional aspect of immunity.

Some people utilize natural cellular encoding for wellness (chapters 1, 2, & 6). By understanding how their cells communicate, analyze, and respond to various stimuli, they harness this knowledge to promote physical and mental well-being. As part of the method to improve cellular function, some people meditate, eat whole and high vibrational foods, and use natural biofeedback practices. Many use natural bioactive compounds and other energies to significantly influence healing and wellness states. Vibrations and frequencies are not limited to the sensory and acoustic realms. Some physicians, registered dieticians, and other practitioners agree that each food, vitamin, and essential oil holds a unique resonance. An accelerometer measures fruit vibrations to determine the firmness of produce. As Albert Einstein stated, "Everything is energy" and "Everything in life is vibration," then, according to the law of vibration, food is energy vibrating at either a high or low frequency. Some scientists describe the benefits of vibrational therapy for use in various medical disciplines.

"Understanding the concept of energy medicine and vibration science in relation to body physiology could provide us with a deeper understanding of the cellular processes that govern healing and perhaps unlock new avenues in tissue engineering." (Beri, 2018). Vibrational wound therapy was shown to help diabetic foot ulcers heal faster. (Syabariyah et al., 2023). In a randomized double-blinded, placebo-controlled clinical trial study, low-magnitude high-frequency vibration improved human balance and muscle strength seen a year after treatment. (Wong et al., 2021). Vibration therapy improved the bone mass in postmenopausal women and the aged. (Singh & Varma, 2023). Some medical professionals believe high-vibrational foods are a vital factor in prevention and the regenerative (healing) process.

Many focus on the fuel (dietary factors) fortifying the immune system and providing energy. Proper cellular metabolism, immune functioning, and stem cell functioning require nutritional support. Fresh vegetables, fruits, herbs, and spices mitigate free radicals, thus inflammation (Jiang et al., 2021), as they chemically instruct human cells to protect the body. Fresh berries, citrus fruits, and celery strengthens human immunity. (Kolarovic et al., 2019).

Researchers have found that certain food constituents may instigate disease. "Dietary proteins {amylase/trypsin inhibitors} can induce inflammation in mice, irritable bowel syndrome, fatty liver disease, and metabolic syndrome." (Dos Santos Guilherme et al., 2020). "A GF diet does not alter normal intestinal microflora; it decreases disease-specific symptoms in those with irritable bowel disease, type 1 and type 2 diabetes, and other medical conditions… and may help prevent them." (Di Liberto et al., 2020). A gluten-free diet can improve triglycerides and cardiovascular health. (Roszkowska et al., 2019).

Other protective considerations involve resveratrol that holds, "anticarcinogenic, antiviral, neuroprotective, anti-inflammatory and antioxidant properties." (Salehi et al., 2018). Resveratrol is a natural component of grapes, red wine, peanuts, and berries. Natural resveratrol and supplements can potentially interact with blood thinners and nonsteroidal anti-inflammatory drugs (NSAIDs), posing a risk for bleeding. This emphasizes the importance of advising all healthcare providers about any natural and supplemental resveratrol, and every prescription and all over-the-counter products you use. Consult your healthcare provider(s) for any questions about this or any other information in this text.

An overlooked constitutive factor of healing is living in the present. Many people spend much of their time thinking about the past or the future, which prevents them from living in this dimension of time. While it is most practical to live in each moment, it is easy to be distracted. Once, I suddenly realized while driving home that I had left my wallet in a grocery basket in the store parking lot. Ater turning around, it was gratefully retrieved intact ten minutes later. When attention is displaced, what was just in our hands can be lost. Constant awareness of what is happening prevents distractions and misplacement.

Living in the present may advance the energy of intentional healing. Implementing these types of measures may seem unfeasible if a provider has set a specific timeline for someone's life. Despite receiving advice to organize their affairs, many patients successfully overcame their disease. This may appear as though only a select few were able to experience a miracle that allowed transmuting biological processes. However, anything experienced by one person must be possible for everyone. At times, another's subjective perception (opinion) may restrict the possibility of that experience. This has occurred as some patients have yielded to the expectations of those in authority. The unique experiences relayed by each cured person contribute to a broader understanding of life itself. When will medical community continue documenting and the research sector examine the common factors underlying these events? Personal and collective perceptions are significant factors that influence the interpretation and response to these events. "Only perception can be sick, because only perception can be wrong." (ACIM, T-8.IX.1:7, p. 158).

Have fixed perceptions perpetuated implicitly accepting limitations of scientific investigations by disregarding certain transparent articles? Research papers throughout this text suggest that personal beliefs can fuel chemical processes, that aid in catalyzing disease. Repetitive thoughts, emotional reactions, and perceptions of current or past emotional and physical traumas are also implicated as disease influencers.

If assessing personal explanations of disease (chapter 6), evaluating specific reasons for healing can aid in understanding expectations. Is the goal to quickly eradicate a disease, or is it to comprehend its symptoms and prevent its recurrence? When my hair shedding appeared excessive, the disruption of the natural order challenged the notion of health certainty as a foundation of truth. This awareness prompted consonance within, shifting focus on how to naturally support my thyroid and adrenals. This encouraged research into strategies for preventing stress, minimizing frequent startles (living in fear and fight-or-flight), and incorporating specific foods. The consistency of these remedies saw a reversal of the symptom.

When can we anticipate comprehensive approaches of intercepting underlying disease mechanisms (chapter 6) and prevention (chapter 7)? Some government supported entities (chapter 5), have documented the psychological (unresolved trauma) and energetic states blocking the normal functioning of specific body organs. These agencies recognize that the grounding of emotions restores wholeness. Most medical communities acknowledge the harmful effects of stress but often overlook the various emotions it can trigger. Though, many researchers acknowledge the virulence of negative emotions stemming from adverse childhood experiences (ACEs) (chapter 6). Can declining to investigate the depth of their findings and those of other government entities contribute to advancing and perpetuating chronic illness?

Many healthcare professionals advise patients that healing certain conditions is improbable or impossible. This statement limits the only outcome to the unlikely or unattainable (bias potentially advancing the nocebo effect). Overlooking disparate data suspends the opportunity to perceive beyond limitations. Some people have reported overcoming medical "certainties" with various energies. Multitudes enhanced probability in different states of consciousness through prayer (meditation and affirmations), allowing a powerful connection with a **higher vibration. A state of invocation or chanting can establish grounding, peace, and direction. Individual and group connection with a divine frequency can be perceived as aligning with the vibration of miracles. In faith believing, some thank a deity for what has already occurred for themselves or others. They see this as activating the particles of matter to assist people simultaneously (quantum superposition).

Those using prayer can doubt or feel disappointed if their healing is not instantaneous or does not occur. When it is believed that a higher power is not granting requests, perhaps the energy was inadvertently being forced. This can prompt anger, uncertainty and disbelief, generating opposition through frustration, and giving up (reaffirming limitations within the feedback loop, inclining lower vibrations). Or, according to Newton's third law of motion: every action or force in nature incurs an equal and opposite reaction (movement in the opposite direction).

Some people infuse spiritual meaning into nature's mathematics via sacred geometry to promote intentional healing through energetic balance and vibratory alignment. The focus on cyclical fractals, perceived as oneness in nature, may synchronize and unify matter for equilibration. Like affirmations, this focus forms new neuropathways or brain rewiring. Many geometric shapes correspond to spherical, cylindrical, and orthogonal structures in the human body. Part of a DNA strand consists of deoxyribose sugar (pentagon shape) mirroring some natural designs. This correspondence, in nature, conveys interconnectedness. Then, nothing is seen as separate from anything else unless it is perceived as so. Quantum entanglement (QE) (equivalent to quantum coherence) occurs when one particle affects another linked particle no matter their distance in space. In separate experiments, scientists Alain Aspect, John Clauser, and Anton Zeilinger won the Nobel Prize for demonstrating QE. Can we then anticipate the authentication of quantum mechanics-based information and non-local healing?

In the meantime, can thermodynamics and quantum biology reverse organ failure? Researchers have studied the thermodynamic analysis of actions, reactions, and interactions in organ dysfunction, as well as the complex communication within organs involving neuro-immune pathways. The acronym (AKI-CKD) refers to acute kidney injury-chronic kidney disease. "Targeting TC (tubular cells) polyploidization after the early AKI phase can prevent AKI-CKD transition without influencing AKI lethality." (De Chiara et al., 2022). Certain nephroprotective plants exhibited antioxidant and anti-inflammatory effects in the hearts and livers of rat models. (Khan et al., 2022). Researchers find that rutin, a flavonoid that is found naturally in citrus fruits and some foods, "has cardioprotective, hepatoprotective, and nephroprotective effects." (Rahmani et al., 2022).

Mental augmentation may include releasing the density of negative emotions (guilt, shame, etc.) and accepting worthiness to allow healing. (ACIM, T-13.X.6:1-6, p. 263). Some scientific articles recognize specific emotions (anger and resentment) as aiding certain disease processes (chapter 6). Some sacred texts describe the benefits of love and peace in healing. Globally, multitudes living in the belief that anything is possible may reside in a higher state of awareness and connection. Can this explain why some research group subjects unknowingly prayed for have experienced healing? The inability to conceptualize anything beyond past experiences influencing beliefs and perception limits potential, enabling one to live within set limitations. When extrapolating the past as indisputable evidence, the logical mind, aligning with collective doubt, can never find a different path.

Diverse questions provide clarity and opportunity for diverse paths. Experiencing different results requires an element of shifting perspective. Perceiving having to change anything can facilitate action or perpetuate inaction. When choosing inaction, one may realize that doing the same things cannot yield different results (Albert Einstein) but find it challenging to overcome a habitual way of being. In a different perspective, one may see the ability to take control of their own mindset and examine current certainties. When individuals recognize their ability to question and alter their long-held convictions, they embark on a transformative path that fosters a deeper understanding of themselves and their circumstances. In the realm of healing, how one decides to continue reacting to an affliction may affect outcomes. Healing can feel separate or unattainable when viewing a disease with anger, resentment, or from a victim's perspective.

Bestowed limitations and countless hospitalizations over her forty-nine earthly years affirmed Barbara as a victim. In my innocence, it was incumbent upon me to be well, as our parents did not need another ill child. That changed in adulthood as emotional trauma surface, prompting conditions requiring medical, surgical, and psychological interventions. I wondered if being a healthy child contributed to Dad's anger, implying I should feel guilty, as his natural daughter was chronically ill. Before the onset of dementia, Dad realized his choice of actions never resolved his emotional density.

Some desired outcomes are planned as athletes and sports teams win competitions by imagining themselves flawlessly completing their moves, being declared winners, or holding medals or trophies. As they love what they do, affirm, visualize, and feel the emotions, they veer toward transcribing their desires. Mental imagery influences emotions (Burnett Heyes et al., 2017) influencing outcomes. There is mutual fulfillment in loving and caring for other people, pets, and plants (all holding unique vibrations). Although all species can detect frequencies differently, humans, livestock, and plants respond to classical music at low decibels. (Cibrorowski et al., 2021) and achieve similar effects. Animal and human immune systems are enhanced by environmental signals. (Ciborowska et al., 2021). Plants, on the other hand, use stimuli to change their cells and metabolism. As prolonged sound exposure can have adverse effects on humans and animals, periods of silence (Cibrorowski et al., 2021) hold their own positive energy.

The vibrational resonance of music can raise vibration and frequency that induces relaxation, feeling good, and love. Autism, obsessive-compulsive disorder, and attention deficit have been treated with dolphin-assisted therapies. (Matamoros et al., 2020). However, some studies have shown that just listening to cetacean frequencies can improve people's mental health. "The up-regulated microRNAs were also found to be regulators of apoptosis, suggesting repression of apoptotic mechanisms in connection with music-performance." (Nair et al., 2019). A study found that classical music exposure to the MCF-7 breast cancer cell line can induce apoptosis (arrest of cellular growth). (Lestard & Capella, 2016). In 2019, Sound Health started researching the effects of music on various medical and mental conditions. (NIH, 2022). Their preliminary findings indicate that music-based therapies are helpful for chronic pain, depression, and anxiety symptoms. (NIH, 2022). Providers selecting an energy to respond disease can consider reviewing these types of studies.

As an antidote to the voice of symptoms representing disease and trauma, some avoid recreating and reliving the same unwanted experiences (chapter 2). Clearing conflict from previously programmed emotional burdens can open a path to living freely in the present. Many find that knowing and living in the perception of their personal truth is integral to intentional healing. Perception shapes the world that one sees (chapter 2). Some medical and mental healthcare providers have not accepted catalyzing healing or sustained well-being through such perceived nonconventional mechanisms, despite a plethora of researcher citations. Einstein's equation $E=MC^2$ posits that energy and matter are interchangeable. Some medical systems see converting energy as influencing mass in the body. If energy and matter are the same, they are interchangeable, and if information is energy, then "the information-energy imbalance of diseases could be corrected." (Wen, 2018). While some still discount this equation as holding human healing potential, many support it by using energy medicine or energy psychology.

As "Everything is energy" (Albert Einstein), energetic healing interventions are being sought. Some seek the evidence-based emotional freedom technique (EFT) (energy psychology) or acupressure point tapping. EFT has been effective in many psychological disorders and physiological conditions. (Church et al., 2022), as it targets underlying emotions. But how can subtle energies such as Qi, Prana, the interactive processes of prayer, and miracles be measured? The Prognos device has been able to check the reliability of acupuncture points along the meridians that carry Qi energy. Studies involving prayer (people perceiving beyond their circumstances) have been performed, and some see the Egely wheel as measuring life energy. Objective and independent researchers can further commit to evaluating unexplainable and spontaneous healings.

In tandem with EFT or other physical and psychological approaches, healing may be found in the power of ***living beyond forgiveness. This act can alleviate physiological stress responses while unforgiveness can raise "heart rate and blood pressure." (Lichtenfeld et al., 2019). According to Akhtar et al. (2017), forgiveness fosters mental well-being and empowers a sense of peace. As anger, hopelessness, fear, and feelings of worthlessness collect, the body can store emotional densities (Chapter 6). As well, automatic reactions to another's words or actions can affect emotional and physical states. Deep breathing can help restore grounding and recalibrate vibratory states to prevent negative reflexes.

Decades ago, my teachers seemed to appreciate the significance of neuroscience. In third grade, a teacher once made me write, "I must not talk in class" 100 times. The purpose of this action was to establish new neural pathways and reinforce the significance of those words, thereby correcting my actions. On lined paper, I wrote, "I must not talk in class" on one side, then only once on the back and all subsequent pages. The rest were ditto marks. When I handed my assignment in, the class watched as the teacher angrily snatched the papers and threw them in the trash. Despite not completing the assignment, it yielded the intended outcome.

Perceiving beyond, medicine may review previous and current neuroscientific findings in consideration of preventing and treating emotional distress. "Choosing to change thoughts helps in being receptive to other sensory information that can produce change." (Rao et al, 2009). Focused attention can induce neuroplasticity (chapter 2). Studies confirm specific brain processes direct desired physiological or behavioral outcomes. Decoded neurofeedback has been effective in ADHD and emotional disorders. (Enriquez-Geppert et al., 2019). Meditative states such as cooking, walking, singing, hobbies, etc., naturally enhance neuroplasticity. Research findings throughout this text may prompt the medical community's curiosity about consciousness-based medicine practices (chapter 9).

In a letter to my surviving sister a couple of years ago, I provided a potential frame of reference regarding her personal ACEs (chapter 6). In her letter, my older sister, who remains ill under current heuristics, was searching for divine help; therefore, my response is largely framed within the spiritual dimension. People assign various names to the supernatural energy that they believe is operating within the universe and their lives. My sister knows this power as God.

Dear Powerful Sister,

Many people believe that healing is a divine promise; however, overcoming professional authoritative opinions can incline fear and doubt. Some clinicians cannot perceive anything beyond the way they have always been or feel bound by limiting standards. Therefore, some people exert their personal authority (power) not by dominating or controlling anything or anyone but by recognizing that which supports their natural ability. Choosing a course of treatment is a joint decision with your qualified licensed healthcare provider(s). Thus, this letter never recommends changing or stopping any prescribed therapy without consulting your doctor. If you have tried everything and have not healed, you may lose confidence in the medical system and the universe. Opening your heart to the power of love and personal truth can restore perceptions of the possible. What you know about yourself is more powerful than what others think or say about you. Limited perceptions continue in the safety and surety of seeing oneself as they already are, rather than what they could be. (ACIM, T-3.IV.2:3-5, p. 42).

You said you are looking for God's help. Do you and God believe that well-being or disease is a natural human state? What is the highest vision you and God can imagine for your life? When prayers seem unanswered, many believe they are forsaken. Though questioning and blaming incline anger and doubt, repelling this level of consciousness, vibration, and frequency* that blocks the cocreation of miracles between divine energy and the divine self. If you have asked for forgiveness-s; it is natural to receive it by forgiving yourself. Some people live beyond forgiveness**** of the past by living in their truth of their identity*** and in self-love, forgoing judgment of themselves, their circumstances, or others.

Judging can block the flow of healing energy and implies fault with creation (yourself and others) and God. There is power in personal truth (**who one knows themselves to be). You are not the lesser thoughts, opinions, or actions of anyone else. No matter what has happened in the past or is happening now, knowing and living in your truth may restore peace in sentient cells. We can choose to live within self-imposed or another's limitations or perceive beyond them.

Disregarding the possible creates a space where only the impossible can exist. Sometimes it seems that only certain people have been able to receive miraculous healing. However, if other people have reversed disease states, including terminal cancer, to wellness, then reversing disease must be a universal human condition.

Then why do some people experience miracles while others do not? Ultimately, the spontaneously healed refused to accept another's authoritative limiting opinions. Many intentionally focused on seeing and feeling their belief as a reality (they existed in what they wanted to experience). Sometimes people may inadvertently counter miracles. Doubt and the emotional load of anger, shame, guilt, resentment, and unworthiness oppose natural healing, as these emotions don't reflect self-love or the ability to accept and receive God's reciprocity of love, light, and healing. Distorted thoughts (illusions) about oneself can create false perceptions, imbuing self-contempt. The habit of focusing on the unwanted amplifies an awareness of negative aspects and cultivates a level of stress and dissatisfaction. Every day, we can see ourselves anew, with symmetry and reverence while reflecting on our personal assets and accomplishments. Some people hold the belief that wholeness or health is not possible when it remains unseen or unfelt, but it can be seen as always existing (according to thermodynamics, p. 125).

Humans can grow up conditioned like baby elephants, knowing the limitations of physical or psychological restraints. This illusion is still perceived as more powerful than the adult elephant's body mass and one's human cognition. Seeing things from a different perspective can change reality. When hospital equipment did not work, the first thing I wanted to know was if it was plugged into its power source. Thus, many people pray alone (personal power) and with a shared intention in an assembly (collective power) to connect with the highest vibration* (Source) some call God consciousness, in the confidence knowing it will be done. Some people pray by and receive by giving thanks for the miracle that has already moved into their **reality. "Whatever you ask for in prayer, believe that you have received it, and it will be yours." (Mark 11:24, KJV). Writing down everything you love in the world and about yourself and focusing on them (Philippians 4:8, KJV) is supported by neuroscience. The journal I sent presents endless possibilities when you write your own story. "I have disowned the truth. Now let me be as faithful in disowning falsity. Whatever suffers is not part of me. What grieves is not myself. What is in pain is but illusion in my mind. What dies was never living in reality and did but mock the truth about myself." (ACIM, W-248.1:1-6, p. 417).

As you know, not everyone who smokes develops a disease. Then what creates the greatest potential for disease? The variable may be the contribution of beliefs creating repetitive, conscious and subconscious thoughts affecting perceptions, emotions, and the physical layer. Some neuroscientific studies show that DNA and negative harmful belief patterns can be overridden by reprogramming or rewiring the brain. This is realized by creating new neuropathways from affirmations, new thoughts and beliefs about oneself, meditation, and visualizations (holographic imagery). The energy of the chemicals created by these actions delivers information to all bodily pathways, allowing new memories to exist and persist.

Every situation presents an opportunity to exert personal authority (power). You can choose not to immediately emotionally react to situations as this can catalyze lower vibrations that support inflammation.

Biophysicist and molecular biologist, Pjotr Garjajev and other researchers assert that DNA responds to words and frequencies, thus can be changed. (Zaja, 2019). People have reversed habits and physical states by changing their thoughts and perceptions about the way things seem to be (unwanted illusions). Some do this by creating and affirming new narratives or beliefs about themselves. These continual thoughts (energy) create new neural pathways, replacing the reinforced beliefs and habits rooted in the previous ways of being. Can you consistently practice being the way you want to be and seeing your desires as already happened? Without limitations, what would you be doing? While everyone wants instant healing, which some have experienced, it cannot be forced. What happened the last time you tried to force anything? The energy of forcing change implies scarcity and separation (ACIM, T-3.V.2:2-4, p. 44) of something, though can be transcended by creating and allowing peace, joy, and unification. (ACIM, T-8.IV.5:4, p. 143).

Some near-death survivors experiencing miracles report their light connected with God's light that flowed curative energy to every human particle, converting emotional pain and physical debilitation to love, light, and peace. Some practitioners see a diseased part separate from the rest of the normally functioning body. However, there is an interconnectedness and interdependence within the structures of the body, and the laws of physics may apply to healing within living systems in that it always exists in **some form. If what is conceivable determines the rules of physics, not the laws themselves, then altering belief allows an activation of a different way.

Many who see themselves as a co-creator with God believe they can transform their circumstances. By not faulting themselves or the past, self-judgment is replaced with self-love.

When placing diagnosed afflictions in perspective, one may see that although a disease is perceived as undesirable, it exists as a part of the body. Therefore, fighting against it implies provoking an opposition within oneself, creating a constant internal conflict that resists healing. However, one may permit the transmutation of disease to its next state of being (by giving it up to God). Alongside shared decisions with a provider, some use various approaches, including but not limited to affirming their beliefs and approaches resonating with their personal beliefs. Words eliciting emotions are powerful in affirming or disclaiming limitations. You can choose to recite personal affirmations with conviction to create new neural pathways (brain rewiring).

Whatever you proclaim, feel it as your truth and see it as already happened. In your imagination, without limitations, what does healing look like and feel like? Affirmations can influence beliefs that can translate into what one knows as truth (chapter 2). With one hand over my heart, the following intention was declared. "I feel every cell in my body responding in oneness with the vibration and frequency* of Divine pure love that permits healing energy and miracles; so be it." Faith is the link connecting the invisible and visible. According to Jesus, healing transpires in faith believing and it is your faith (belief) that heals. (Mark 5:34, KJV).

The first law of thermodynamics posits that energy is neither created nor destroyed; it only changes form. This law permits the transmission of energy between locations to change forms. Thus, a system and its surroundings can exchange the highest energy particles without direct contact. In the context of healing, this principle suggests that the energy within the body is conserved and can be redirected or converted to another form. This understanding facilitates the exploration of healing approaches that align with the natural principles governing energy. If nothing is created or destroyed, then everything including healing energy** has always existed in some form. And healing is always possible as everything exists simultaneously; therefore, healing can be seen as always being available to be transformed into reality. But then, under this law, all negative things (the unwanted past and disease) will always exist and cannot be destroyed. Yes, but according to this law, their energy can be transformed. As disease disrupts information pathways required for the flow of energy, you can decide to reconnect to the restorative energies, chapter 11, and release disease/symptoms to the light of God.

Nikola Tesla said, "If you want to find the secrets of the universe, think in terms of energy, frequency, and vibration." Albert Einstein stated, "Everything in life is vibration" and "Everything is energy, and that's all there is to it. Match the frequency of the reality you want, and you cannot help but get that reality. It can be no other way. This is not philosophy, this is physics." Did inventors perceive these statements as a framework for moving their ideas and desires into existence? Did they transcend beyond collective limited perceptions through their imaginations that created a pathway toward a certain reality? Were the words of an engineer and theoretical physicist the commanding structures solidifying the knowing of an existence of a dimension beyond their current level of understanding; as according to thermodynamics, everything exists in some form? Some believe that according to Einstein, the energy of the vibration and frequency of an inventor or the sick can connect to and match the Divine Inventor's and Divine Healer's to reach their desired reality. Thus, the response received can reflect the type of vibrational signal humans send.

Everything was imagined before it came into existence. Then, can healing be possible by shifting the cellular processes through imagination and visualization, and guided imagery? Do you believe that anything, even a miracle, is possible? "Miracles occur naturally as expressions of love. The real miracle is the love that inspires them. In this sense, everything that comes from love is a miracle." (ACIM, T-1.I.3:1-3, p. 3). Many see prayer as a driving force (energy) that draws limitless potential and miracles into the physical world. When immersed in the energy of prayer (meditation), confident focus (consciousness) can trigger the energy (power) to connect to anything. People can accept and receive the miracle when they perceive the extraordinary with confidence, without doubt, but by knowing it has already occurred. Many refute the ability to co-create with a god or that a high vibration and frequency can enable healing, and this mechanism can be perceived as self-healing.

However, thoughts, beliefs, and perceptions influence feelings, vibration and frequency, thus personal reality (chapter 2). Beliefs are not always facts; they are repetitive thoughts we have accepted as truth. The thought of challenging them can be seen as difficult since they are deeply woven into our identity, emotions, and worldview. However, choosing to challenge beliefs helps in becoming open to a new way of thinking and perhaps a new reality.

In consistent hyperawareness of being cured, one can only know themselves as nothing else but what they are. Then why do some diseased then cured people experience the return of a disease? If the findings of Albert Einstein and Nikola Tesla extend to the human system, then the strengthening of personal truth, love, and peace can lead to higher vibrations and frequencies to connect with desires. Negative emotions in the continual feedback loop of unfavorable thoughts and feelings can effectuate imbalance, misalignment, and disharmony, allowing the grounding and reemergence of the same or another disease. Is it possible that people can choose to see healing as the only possible way things could be?

Without examining me, one physician predicted I would only regain 50% of functioning after a surgical procedure. While some may have assimilated this authoritative statement into their reality, power was demonstrated by refusing to accept their opinion. I am now fully recovered. Without defining an underlying cause of my then persistent postsurgical pain, persuasion was used to coax me into using a regimen with known irreversible side effects. The doctor did not see repetitively asking me why I didn't want to resolve my pain as violating tenets of clinical ethics. I then found myself in the position of a dissatisfied patient and on my own.

Multifunctional applications, including energy practices, may have allowed transmuting the previous memory patterns (ways of being) of pain and dysfunction. The techniques I applied demonstrated heart over mind, not mind over matter (Sobolewska-Nowak et al., 2023).

Are you open to perceiving things in a different way? Researchers and Scripture suggest that a change in perception and love transcends everything. A friend of mine said they could only see something on its face. I replied, "Then we would never have gone to the moon or currently enjoy all the advances of those who had perceived beyond." Confirmation bias (believing there is only one certain way things can be) can keep us confined to our current way of being.

You may wonder if you have prayed why, it is that healing was delayed or didn't happen. You may have been devout in prayer and felt disappointment inclining doubt. If believing that a higher power is not fulfilling requests, it could be due to unintentionally forcing energy. Demanding an action can prompt feelings of anger, uncertainty, and disbelief, generating opposition through frustration, and giving up (reaffirming limitations within the feedback loop, inclining lower vibrations and frequencies). Or, according to Newton's third law of motion: every action or force in nature incurs an equal and opposite reaction (movement in the opposite direction).

If able, intentional, slow, deep breaths provide grounding. In this energy, there is an opportunity to revisit the fundamental beliefs shaping your emotions and the perceptions that shape your truth. Many believe that free will (the ability to choose beliefs) is powerful in creating personal destiny. Ultimately, you choose your beliefs, your truth.

Your loving sister

The next chapter explores the potential advancements in healthcare and inquiries surrounding medical ethics. Can clinicians continue accepting any ineffective operational methods or collaborate on their visions for an improved healthcare system?

# Chapter 9

## Informing the Future of Healthcare

**"The doctor of the future will give no medicine but will interest his patient in the cure of the human frame, in diet and in the cause and prevention of disease."  ~ Thomas Edison**

**"Many medical schools inform their students that within several years half of what they've been taught will be wrong, and the teachers just don't know which half."  ~ Samuel Arbesman**

**"A prevailing theory or paradigm is not overthrown by the accumulation of contrary evidence," "but rather by a new paradigm that, for whatever reasons, begins to be accepted by scientists."  ~ Richard Zeckhauser**

**"The medicine of the future will be frequency medicine."**
~ Albert Einstein

The challenge is on for the most revolutionary presentation of a safe, efficient, and cost-effective healthcare system. How will contestants answer the societal discontent of perceived ubiquitous care models? Will medical consumers' concerns be perceived as a threat to routine patterns or as an opportunity to enhance the quality of healthcare service? Can contestants aptly identify the risks versus benefits of proposed change versus inaction? Appraising the ends of medicine in regard to suffering humans deserves an immediate response. Assessing a broad sample of consumer responses about the output of medicine, reflecting the sectors responsible for care, defines the next step. No objections may imply satisfaction, while grievances direct the concerned and curious to investigate each complaint. If medical consumer surveys asked open-ended questions that accurately captured patient perceptions their satisfaction with healing, what insights would emerge?

If the competitors of healthcare improvement identify the need for actual care based on patient value, will it be framed in amending or overhauling the current paradigm? Do proposed archetypes consider improvements that satisfy consumers' vision to avert the enormity of future social affronts? Despite the many decades of government and independent agency identification of the market issues and recommendations for a more efficacious health system, progress could be faster. What individual or team can build upon this momentum for desired clinician and consumer change (chapter 5)? And overcome perceived healthcare predicaments for professional and consumer confidence in the medical product? Which model systematically can perceive equitability to payers and providers that serves consumers?

Working amid perpetual unresolved issues can prompt clinicians to appeal to their influential professional associations for review. Lobbying professional and government entities represents the value of every human life. If there is little or no response after following up on human concerns and burdens, new associations and organizations may close the gap of addressing creditable clinician and patient distresses. This may mobilize professional organizations and public healthcare institutions to take note of biomedical researchers' concerns and reevaluate current research methodology. Providers can assist those developing a payer prospectus by reviewing the most transparent research conclusions that demonstrate the healthcare system's ability to achieve effective outcomes. Free information from government websites and the Freedom of Information Act (available in many countries) can be used to obtain and review current and ongoing research information. Healthcare communities, professionals, and organizations can benefit humanity by reevaluating the functionality of their medical system.

Will professional duty prompt taking the first step toward assessing a possible colossal paradigm shift? Bringing anything, including a potential new medical model, into reality involves overcoming perceived obstacles. Without imposing limitations or doubt, what is the highest expectation a clinician can perceive for each patient experiencing suffering? Throughout recorded history, a lack of vision has caused death and destruction. "The only thing worse than being blind is having sight but no vision." (Helen Keller). Can those attempting to improve a medical system imagine how the ultimate care model might look from all vantage points?

Can clinicians imagine a future that includes the now uncommon endocrine, heart, neurological, and other disease states and disorders as root causes were fully addressed? Understanding the primary source(s) of disease assures accurate corrective and preventative measures. It is then that clinicians and consumers can realize the full intention of the medical product. This success would increase the need for many more contemporized healthcare professionals to support consumers in reaching wellness states.

Those looking to create a unified conceptual model of healing, health, and wellness maintenance can commit to being in the energy of solutions, not in perpetuation of the problem. The greatest achievements for humanity were resolved by posing the purest questions (curiosity without preconceived expectations) for the most unbiased answers. Viewing situations from multiple points of view helps refocus tunnel vision. This may help to evaluate efficacious versus ineffective measures Since the foundation of medical practice relies on impeccable research practices, does a new perspective consider a thorough review of data designated to support current evidence-based medicine practices (EBM)?

This action filters down to other medical entities, like those reviewing biomedical papers for translation of quality interventions for clinical application. As a cross-check, will translation services be entitled to discern the journey of scientific conclusions in the perspective of objectivity, openness, and transparency before dissemination for implementation? Awareness and mitigation of research issues (chapter 3) can assist in delivering a more precise health communication model. Then all medical entities considering transparent articles can review diverse data for potential application of the least effort to enhance natural capacity and desired outcomes. These precise actions may help avoid overmedicalization, a premise of quaternary prevention. Attention to biomedical papers overcoming obstacles experienced in the scientific research arena translates to better healthcare delivery and genuine realization of the intended product. Otherwise, health insurance payers may structure payments to reflect their knowledge and interpretation of the fundamentals of current EBM practice. Specifically, regarding unresolved issues within the investigative process, overlooked transparent research findings, and confirmed healing successes or dismissed and unimplemented curatives.

Can payers ever hold practitioners, medical organizations, and policy-makers accountable for not pursuing or instituting all available effective and affordable interventions? As insurers understand the medical ethics mandate of all healthcare entities, they can act in the best interest of their subscribers. This commitment can enhance the research article review method (chapter 3) to analyze biomedical researchers' findings of correct diagnostics and disease pathology influencing therapeutic and preventative approaches. Comparing current interventions to open and transparent biomedical research papers and lifestyle clinics' evidential findings for safety, effectiveness, and overall cost of interventions helps substantiate a rational foundation of healing and wellness. This action may encourage insurers to lobby their government and professional organizations to affect policymaking favorably.

Insurers may interpret harm as occurring from many types of interventions and see the future of medicine remaining accountable to the quality of the research enterprise. If payers evaluated if harm was preventable, could they view a medical system as accountable? Will they recognize and cover complementary and alternative medicine (CAM) within a review of diverse researchers' and potential new parameters (Chapter 5) of the National Center for Complementary and Integrative Health (NCCIH)? Highly regarded institutes pursued CAM research as the world expressed disenfranchisement with healing results. Did the perception of folk sector empowerment prompt the NCCIH to respond by expanding CAM therapy research. (NCCIH, 2023)? Clinicians can assess the journey of clinical trials (research competence) (Chapter 3) currently underway in potential disease prevention and treatment considerations for informed CAM decision-making. Will recommendations consider examining research in psychiatry and the effectiveness of a multi-perspective approach?

Will those in a new perception of multi-faceted human beings revisit biopsychosocial dimensions confirmed by that many researchers? As a medical system universally defines health and disease, stakeholder cooperation of how stewardship is structured and incentivized can help clinicians deliver high-value care. This requires a new vision to build upon the strengths of a healthcare system while recognizing where the current operations of medicine fall short.

In past centuries, homeopathy was recognized by Western Medicine (WM) as a basic healing method. As perceptions of this approach have continually changed, will the future come full circle to its past? How previous biomedical investigations were performed and selected for standards has led medicine to this point. Investigating confirmed and unexplained successes can help advance the goal of biomedical research and the medical field. The clarity of correct disease determinants leading to lasting correction will restore truth in medicine as practitioners consistently respond to clients beyond symptom management. In this perspective, a case for a paradigm shift based on a patients' desire for freedom from suffering can be made. Medicine can best serve consumers by becoming proactive and shifting to more preventative, health, and wellness-focused programs instead of practicing reaction medicine Have all concerns of those using the healthcare system been attained, understood, and respected (Chapter 5)? Via surveys, what have providers and organizations learned from assessing patient perspectives of the functionality of their current system? Dismissing contrasting views has already driven patients to consult the Internet, a medical intuitive, channeler, and other self-healing guidance. Are you a clinician researching or using other healing methods?

Medical consumers who perceive receiving fragmented care are continuing to find a way to transmute the imbalances of illness to wellness. Some are consulting social media, CAM practitioners, integrative care or indigenous providers, and spiritual leaders. Increasingly, people are being drawn to the perceived benefits of acupressure and massage in prevention and anticipation of restoration of harmony and balance. Many are seeking yoga, tai chi, music, dance, Reiki, Qigong, and a higher awareness* for disease prevention and healing. Some perceive the benefits of other energy medicines like the confirmed psychological and physiological effects of the Emotional Freedom Technique (Chapter 8), that interrupts thought patterns. This can provide a foundation for integrating neuroscientific findings in disease prevention and treatment. Paired stimuli-reward inclining attention is associated with automatic remembering affecting future rewards. (Tibboel & Liefooghe, 2020). The more personal value one receives from an intervention, the more it will be sought.

The following personal axioms envision how WM will likely look in the foreseeable future. As more autobiographies describe personal experiences with telepathic communication, the unexplainable, and miraculous, the public's interest heightens. As medicine supports longitudinal, cross-sectional, and other study methodology, they identify the mechanisms of spontaneous remissions. Telemedicine services will increase and prioritize prevention. Provider offices are expected to expand into lifestyle clinics in the fashion of Dr. Dean Ornish and beyond** to focus on proactive medicine and effectuate healing. These clinics will inform clients about the applications of new body monitors and devices. Consumers can perceive value in these types of comprehensive outpatient wellness clinics* that will multiply exponentially. As these above and beyond clinics follow scientific models viewing humans as multifaceted conscious beings, maximum potential advances via expert interdisciplinary teams. By looking beyond limitations, practitioners in these clinics will consider the various multidimensional factors involved in disease pathology, as detailed in all chapters, to effectively address chronic disease.

One technique that will be offered in these transformative clinics is education on consciousness-based medicine** and how to move desired energy into reality (chapters 2, 5 & 8). This will also involve the reprogramming of memory engrams (chapters 2 & 6) to heal chronic diseases including cancer. Transparent research will report that people living in the energies of peace and harmony within themselves (at a higher vibration and frequency), can help mitigate disease. The field of organ and tissue regenerative engineering (Ajmal et al., 2023) expands as nanotechnology and medical engineering methods are perfected. Scientific research will extend to discovering self-regulatory mechanisms of biological processes. This dispels the illusion that only certain people can survive firewalking, being submerged in frigid waters like magicians, or control their vital signs like focused monks.

Researchers will disclose the chemical processes and neurocognitive components that allow self-thermoregulation, potentially by g-tummo meditation. (Kozhevnikov et al., 2013) or other mind-body techniques for prevention and therapeutic intervention. Full-service medical clinics and primary care provider offices known as whole-person resource clinics* and substance abuse centers will consider offering several verifiable options. Clients can choose from epigenetic guidance, guided imagery, conscious living, consciousness-based medicine interventions, and counseling to understand the nature of self-actualization and transcendence. Then, medical and specialty providers and programs will be inundated with medical consumers seeking to integrate all aspects of their multidimensional selves and realize their enlightenment. Usage of a medical system producing desired results demands a fully staffed expert workforce. Provider offices choosing not to engage in whole-person services then can make specialty referrals (the collaborative care model) without perceiving professional rivalry.

Examining disparate biomedical researchers' discoveries supplies providers with a clear path to shift from palliative care (symptom relief) to consistent solutions. A novel paradigm that targets the fundamental causes of disease and disorders spurs the creation of multifaceted evaluations for disease prevention and focused interventions. When this responsibility is met, medical professionals will no longer be positioned to practice defensive medicine. Medical workers will have an opportunity to live in the confidence of the mission, vision, and value statements of their institutions and professional associations. As clinicians, medical workers, and patients hold the highest perspective and vision for healing and cure, they can be better realized.

Competition in the health insurance industry can increase if more hospital centers consider offering health coverage that expands services that address all human dimensions. The demand for these insurers can increase if coverage extends to out-of-network providers. Practitioners offering a more value-perceived-based care approach will have considered open and transparent biomedical researchers' successes. This action may prompt them to lobby organizations for the reevaluation of current standards to improve healthcare industry output (care). Especially when the institution's own transparent biomedical study conclusions replicate existing studies establishing healing within a comprehensive whole-person approach. These advanced medical centers can then offer, employ, and cover various care providers (physician specialists, mental health professionals, spiritual liaisons, CAM practitioners, and specialty programs, etc.).

After a comprehensive review of transparent research papers, an extensive EBM reference manual may define causal nexuses to accurately assess and correct disease determinates. Some medical systems (chapter 5) have recognized how emotions and unresolved trauma can catalyze disease and have refined their care approaches accordingly. If this archetype is accepted by WM, medical care could expand. There would be a greater need for more mental health and trauma (post-traumatic stress disorder) (PTSD) interventionists assessing and treating emotional distresses and PTSD diagnoses found to affect the physical layer. Many more books and biomedical article authors, and medical seminar hosts detailing a multi-leveled healing approach in reaching the goal of healthcare will follow this text.

Legal implications can apply if medical professionals observing medical system norms advise patients to follow recommendations which then cause harm (chapter 5). The concept of seeing people as a whole and investigating root causes of disease has been around for decades. However, most commercial funding commitments favor the continuation of the same line and methods of research. Expanding research based on medical consumers' expectations of cure respects the existence of every human life and the practice of medicine. Can patient expectations work together with the goals of medicine to find a path of least resistance without biases to create positive differences? That is, will a medical system that offers measures necessary to human survival opt to perform various kinds of scientific research in search of curative solutions?

Will the public's immeasurable dissatisfaction be what presses change? Community resistance was demonstrated long ago by consulting other healing venues to address personal suffering. Delivering healthcare services based on the same research questions, experiments, and partiality will inevitably lead to the same results. Lay people finding treatments or cures for their loved ones' rare diseases (chapter 6) realized that verity. As well, providers performing their own in-depth investigations and analyses of the scientific literature, consulting with colleagues who are doing the same can inform their professional associations.

Health care environments insinuate a balance between consumer expectations of medicine and economic transaction. However, this is not necessarily perceived as so. Is a medical system remiss due to selective perception by dismissing those who have reversed common and chronic diseases (including terminal cancer) (chapter 8)? Does a business offering healing measures have an obligation to sincerely review such cases and attempt to identify solutions that may prove to be consistently effective? Can the actions of those operating within a medical system be justifiable if numerous replicated biomedical research articles supporting effective healing disparate from current standards were disregarded? If recognition of the decades of scientific biomedical papers addressing the need to see a person as a whole being was regarded, would it have averted the perception of omission? Many more biomedical investigators than cited within this text have established the interconnectedness of the mind-body connection and its relation to disease. What could happen if medical communities and health organizations consistently disregarded patients and researchers concerns about what is found to be harmful or efficacious? As well, are the biomedical researchers' findings in other countries being vetted, considered, or recognized? Could state advocates representing concerned populations take class action?

What if the public's legal counsel established evidence to confirm that damages (pain, suffering, and loss) were caused by preventable breaches of medical system duty? Despite existing standards, if care compromises ethical standards of "justice, beneficence, nonmaleficence, and autonomy" (Mousavi, 2024) (chapter 5), will practitioners need to provide patients with every available option for informed shared decision-making to prevent harm? Could reasonable doubt be established if standard actions and how they were determined deviated from those of similar medical systems, their own standards, and international regulatory standards? Even if they did not deviate, was there an assessment of those standards as being impeccable or substandard? Did providers, professional and health organizations, and policymakers fail to reevaluate the foundation for care (transparent research) and act to change ineffective standards and establish efficient ones? Is continuing to ignore potentially flawed evidence (chapter 3) establishing standards and not taking appropriate action negligent? If providers and medical consumers reported certain standards as consistently unsafe, harmful (chapter 5), or non-efficacious, and these concerns were dismissed, can there be legal recourse?

Can professional organizations' documents, articles, missions, values, and other statements establishing what current and future medical providers should be doing be seen as inaction if they were not standardized or followed? Could collective perceptions be that all avenues toward health freedoms were not pursued? Had the medical field taken appropriate action in correcting research issues influencing guidelines, would harm have not occurred? Avoiding legal issues is not the only impetus to support medical ethics. In preventing harm to human beings, investigating every aspect of curing them as the collective incentive relieves the consumer burden of having to overcome a medical system's imperfections (Introduction).

Quantum communication is expected to optimize workforce, healthcare, and global challenges, leading to improving outcomes for humanity. Programmers will ensure that the output quality from these advanced systems aligns with the responsible embedding of their programming. Researchers will resolve research issues to maintain the integrity of science. These enhancements will empower providers to make decisions from an expanded inventory of possibilities, not from limitations. Clinicians can envision a new or improved healthcare design that enhances educational and clinical structures, enabling an expectation of consistent and effective outcomes. The commitments of the biomedical research and energy sectors are expected to help resolve issues for favorable shifts in healthcare, ecology, and beyond.

# Chapter 10

## Powerful Connections

"A human being is a part of the whole called by us universe, a part limited in time and space. He experiences himself, his thoughts and feeling as something separated from the rest, a kind of optical delusion of his consciousness. This delusion is a kind of prison for us, restricting us to our personal desires and to affection for a few persons nearest to us. Our task must be to free ourselves from this prison by widening our circle of compassion to embrace all living creatures and the whole of nature in its beauty." ~ Albert Einstein

"In our quest for happiness and the avoidance of suffering, we are all fundamentally the same, and therefore equal. Despite the characteristics that differentiate us - race, language, religion, gender, wealth and many others - we are all equal in terms of our basic humanity." ~ Dalai Lama

**"And you might define the ethnosphere as being the sum total of all the thoughts, dreams, ideals, myths, intuitions, and inspirations brought into being by the imagination since the dawn of consciousness." ~ Wade Davis**

Have you ever felt awkward when meeting someone for the first time? This personal experience is shared as it applies to any situation triggering intense emotions requiring personal strength. Upon introduction to someone joining our group, instead of exchanging pleasantries, an unexpected comment was made. Consuming my smoothie through a straw had prompted the remark. This act immediately triggered offense, separation, and perhaps untoward physiological changes in the other person.

While people feel connected to marine animals and don't want to see them become entangled in, injured, or die from human-caused environmental impacts (pollution from ocean plastics), reflex reactions can hamper personal interests. The love for animals may have generated an automated response to an emotional trigger; however, it overshadowed a teaching moment. An objective perspective may have seen that a plastic straw can be recycled within a larger recyclable container. The establishment could have been asked to consider offering reusable straws, encouraging customers to bring their own reusable ones, or providing an area for cleaning and a large plastic container for depositing and recycling them.

As the exchange concluded, maintaining personal power meant not matching another's vibrations and respecting their convictions without passing judgment or embarrassing them. Being an advocate for something can have a greater impact, as the energy of being against anything can invoke opposition, pushback, and argument. Those connected to the environment can support it by taking advantage of educational opportunities and getting involved in causes that shape the type of world they desire to live in. "Be the change that you wish to see in the world." (Mahama Gandhi), serves as a powerful reminder that individual action can ignite broader societal transformation. The expression of an individual's benevolence is an invaluable contributor to the planet's wellness.

Because I feel a connection to the planet, I always recycle. This connection contributes to conserving energy and preventing pollution. People are more likely to recycle if they perceive value in their actions (how they will benefit society). If you're new to recycling, local waste disposal websites and these stations post items accepted at recycling centers. Generally, recycling centers accept paper, cardboard, rinsed and dry cans, glass, and plastic bottles. Specific eco-friendly centers typically accept plastic clamshells, berry and salad containers, and plastic wrapping around products. Within the United States (U.S.), the search.earth911.com database and 1800 cleanup phone number provide complete information about recycling.

Recyclables (clothes, jewelry, and household items) donated or bequeathed prevents them from ending up in landfills. This effort helps prevent the production and buildup of methane gas, carbon dioxide, and ammonia (landfill gases). "Landfill leachate forms when water seeps through waste and undergoes biochemical transformation." (Torres-González et al., 2021). Chemicals drawn out from that waste can contaminate groundwater (drinking water). (EPA, 2023). In the United States, 16% of energy projects have captured and converted landfill gases to renewable natural gas, and more than half of these operations generate electricity. (EPA, 2023). Damage occurs when ammonia produces nitrate and eutrophication (lack of oxygen), creating dead zones, and eradicating animal habitats. (National Ocean Service (NOS), 2023). The global number of oceanic dead zones (where little or no dissolved oxygen exists) has increased. (NOS, 2023). This has reduced plankton (food) for some whales, other marine life, and half of the planet's oxygen supply. (NOS, 2023). Although national and international groups restore marine habitats, voluntary engagement in or support of global ocean cleaning efforts sustains current and future ways of life. This action contributes to protecting the major portion of the world's sea life and significant oxygen production.

Human connection to all living systems encourages caring for the Earth. Planetary health includes mitigating human actions that degrade the natural environment; thus, preventing disease extends to preserving ecosystems and biodiversity (all living things) (Prescott et al., 2019). To prevent and minimize ecosystem damage, healthcare professionals can educate the public not to flush or throw hazardous items away. Local waste management centers guide the proper disposal of batteries, electronic equipment, paint, household cleaners, and other chemicals. Human actions can mitigate the acquired and natural degradation of environments, thereby preventing the extinction of organisms. This awareness can prevent the decline of ecosystems and restore health and the quality of life through the structure and function of human and animal necessities. This consciousness can prompt actions to renew the natural ecological community (thousands of interconnected organisms), living and non-living components interacting with their environment. This helps the landscape and biosphere, influencing the Earth's physical and chemical properties.

Coexistence is achieved by recognizing and addressing the needs of other species and their environments. This perception helps prevent species from endangerment and extinction from habitat loss, pollution, and overharvesting. Interrupting poaching can prevent the depletion of whales and other marine life, which disrupts ecosystem stability and planetary balance. Everyone can check their government wildlife accountability office website for their current studies and recommendations.

Are environmental challenges viewed as an indomitable obstacle or an opportunity for revitalization? As this chapter continues bringing awareness to issues affecting everyone, the perspective of shared solutions generates pure questions. Ecology can benefit from challenging norms and paradigms yielding the same responses. Highlighting global concerns encourages the energy of a vision veering toward the possible.

An awareness of global mining can reduce loss of biodiversity, soil erosion, surface water contamination, and sinkholes. (Stewart, 2020). Attention to this issue can prevent accidents, dust, toxins, stress, and the emergence of diseases in workers and local populations (Stewart, 2020). There is an increased demand for extraction of metal resources for batteries. Batteries must be manufactured as recyclable. (Hantanasirisakul & Sawangphruk, 2023). This perception can prevent batteries and other energy devices like solar panels, from ending up in landfills.

Researchers are attempting to overcome multiple objections while meeting growing global energy demands. As they weigh technological progress objectives with renewable energy technologies, they must account for human and animal health, safety, and environmental impact. Challenges include threats to wildlife from wind turbines, solar panel manufacturing that produces greenhouse gas emissions, and intermittent power production from the above energy devices. (Chatterjee & Dethlefs, 2022). Will manufacturers consider making future energy devices smaller and more efficient? As the research and energy sectors weigh the pros and cons of supporting large-scale battery use and recharging efforts, they hold mixed reactions.

When purchasing products requiring batteries, people are unaware they may be supporting child labor, which is found throughout the Democratic Republic of the Congo and in the Copperbelt region. (U.S. Department of Labor). The latter area accounts for most of the world's cobalt mining and refinement. (U.S. Department of Labor). Global awareness of over-mining of the geosphere (minerals, metals, gemstones), deforestation, urbanization (affecting natural habitats), and overharvesting can help inspire the efforts to restore natural balance.

Urbanization leading to degradation of forests is associated with higher vector-borne pathogen transmission in Central America. (Ortiz et al., 2021) and loss of animal habitat. Because the planet is interconnected, what happens in one place can occur in another. Many human gestures can work to favorably shift from local levels to a global scale. Every year, on the last Friday in April, our grade school commemorated Arbor Day by planting a new seedling. Observing this purposeful act helped me appreciate and connect to trees and nature. On a larger scale, everyone can be stewards of forests through the awareness of each United States' proactive Forest Action Plan. The United Nations (UN) Global Forest Goals promotes sustainable global land and forest management by 2030. (UN, 2018). Although some global forestry plans are voluntary, having constituents undersign can strengthen the verbal commitments of Member States.

People may not be aware of multilevel conservation efforts nor their relevance. Though crops and plants rely on nitrogen and phosphorus for nutrients, too much can pollute the groundwater (Wang & Huang, 2021). Pesticide and fertilizer runoff affect algae growth, blocking sunlight thus, depleting water's oxygen capacity (Kazmi et al., 2022). While methods for removing these elements from water exist (Li et al., 2022), individuals can take further action to reduce adding to the issue to maintain ecological balance. Simple acts like cleaning up and disposing of pet waste and choosing phosphate-free cleaning products (safer choice label). (EPA, 2022) help stop water pollution. Worldwide usage of non-toxic cleaning materials and natural personal products reduces bodily and planetary contamination. Public influence is exerted by choosing non-toxic products, making them at home (recipes at EPA.gov), and urging manufacturers to produce them.

The 2020 pandemic mandates that required humans and pets to spend time indoors inadvertently posed other health risks. There was extended exposure to air pollutants from mold, chemicals, vapors, allergens, lead, formaldehyde, and radon. Mitigating radon (EPA, 2023), may prevent disease and exacerbation of existing conditions. Multilayered indoor air filters, antibacterial, and HEPA filters may help. Preventing toxicity in food, air, and water supplies limits passing toxins to animals, plants, and generationally.

Our relationship with the Earth has significant implications for protecting resources and all species. As human, animal, and plant lives continue to intersect, the bond between species and Earth's elements seeks balance. National and international ocean cleaning efforts are successful in mitigating plastic and microplastics in the Great Pacific Garbage Patch (the size of Texas floating between Hawaii and California). Some organizations continue working to conserve and restore marine habitats and protect the world's significant oxygen production. Everyone can help by being aware of personal choices and actions.

Some strategies require international cooperative efforts in producing safe biodegradable plastics, deposit-refund programs (Prata et al., 2019), and public education programs. Eco-wise companies help by making and selling clothing, footwear, reusable bags, and jewelry made from recycled plastics. Some clothing items partially made from plastic may sound familiar (polyester, nylon, and acrylic). Clothing and plastics made from polyethylene terephthalate (PET) can cause pollution, endangering ecosystems and human health (Soong et al., 2022). As current methods of recycling PET can lead to leaching, sustaining the plastic industry may hinge on correct biodegradation strategies. (Soong et al., 2022).

Other chemicals (Benzothiazole) can penetrate skin layers, causing human health conditions. Bisphenol A (BPA) is found in some medical devices and common consumer products. All species are at risk of health issues and potential extinction due to chemicals, pesticides, and erosion. Some government agency websites list chemicals that can cause adverse human effects, including those that disrupt the endocrine system, in their fact sheets (Chapter 6). Chemicals can interfere with hormonal and cellular functioning and impair immune functioning predisposing humans and animals to diseases. Heavy metals and endocrine-disrupting chemical (EDC) compounds in microplastics and nanoplastics put marine and human life at risk (Ullah et al., 2023). "Recent studies showed a link between EDC exposure with obesity, metabolic syndrome, and type 2 diabetes." (Guarnotta et al., 2022).

Persistent organic pollutants (POPs) are toxic chemicals that break down slowly and can enter the air and water, negatively impacting human and wildlife populations worldwide. The POPs (pesticides and industrial chemicals) accumulate in adipose tissue and disrupt endocrine functioning (Barrett, 2013), contributing to the development of type 2 diabetes. (Lee et al., 2018). The UN encourages countries to create policies and practices in protecting ecosystems from further degradation. Signatories of the UN Treaty or Stockholm Convention say they are active in reducing or eliminating POPs. In 2001, the International UN Millennium Ecosystem Assessment appraised the world's ecological conditions. Their findings, released in 2005, and their technical assessment in 2006 included increased degradation in ecosystems due to food, water, timber, fiber, and fuel demands. They have encouraged nearly every country to follow recommendations to decrease and reverse degradation. However, not all governments have seriously regarded the impact, nor are they taking recommended actions. Therefore, they should encourage signed government treaties to include a monitoring and enforcement clause to make them more meaningful. Otherwise, the degradation and exploitation of biodiversity will persist.

Global awareness of the magnitude and impact of wildlife crime can reduce or eliminate the demand for products. Crimes against wildlife include poaching and trafficking of many animals, including coral, wild flora and fauna, and rosewood. (United Nations Office on Drugs and Crime, World Wildlife Report, 2020). Global awareness underscores the need for action, given that suspected traffickers originate from over 150 countries. Although ivory and pangolin regulations have tightened, wildlife market crimes continue. There were reports of aerial surveillance halted poaching of Mozambique's elephant population in Niassa National Reserve in 2019. However, crimes against wild animals continue. Compiling seizure data (illegal trade reporting) is vital in stopping these crimes and may help save protected species. Not purchasing or consuming illegally poached or transported products as a tourist or consumer can decrease poaching.

The World WISE Database shows the seizure of over 6,000 species of mammals, reptiles, corals, birds, and fish, from 1999 to 2018. Since poaching occurs in every country, global concern can recognize the illegal harvesting of wildlife as a wildlife crime. The international public can check if their country holds sanctions for these actions. Eight percent of the 8,3000 known animal breeds are extinct, and 22% are at risk. (World Wise). Although zoos and wildlife sanctuaries help endangered species, animals are not naturally living wild. Countries committed to addressing root issues may help wildlife live free and unendangered. Governments and citizens can perceive the value in the actions required for tourists to safely view animals in their natural habitats.

Human trafficking is also of great international concern, affecting everyone. In the U.S., providers suspecting or knowing of any trafficked and/or abused person are required to contact child protective services for minors (under 18) and law enforcement (911 in the U.S., and the confidential National

Human Trafficking Hotline (U.S.) at 1-888-373-7888. Worldwide, healthcare professionals can check their country's requirements and contact information for reporting emergencies, abuse, human trafficking, and other crimes. National and international government and outreach websites guide health professionals on how to assist human trafficking victims and products that likely support forced child labor.

Many people are focusing on maximizing future energy needs however, first, it is necessary to perceive it as realizable. Multi-perspectivity prevents seeing things just one way (tunnel vision). Some cities have weighed the positive and negative impact of Smart Grid technology, even as they currently employ specific energy-efficient solutions. Microbial biotechnology producing biofuels (Ramamurthy et al., 2021), and renewable natural gas (from landfills, organic wastes, etcetera) (EPA, 2020), can power vehicles. The first law of thermodynamics or the law of conservation (Chapter 8) states that nothing creates or destroys, implying that everything already exists. From a different perspective, did Nikola Tesla and other inventors' sudden inspirations possibly have connected them to existing information?

Some wonder about further investigation of Nikola Tesla's wireless power technology and the role of artificial intelligence (AI) within the energy sector. Those concerned about harm from electromagnetic fields (EMFs) may see science revisiting Tesla's experiments to create a unified theory of safely containing all EMFs. "The good outcomes seen here show that the quasi-optical framework is helpful for creating highly efficient radiative wireless power transfer systems." (Pereira & Carvalho, 2022). The energy sector can present challenges to the public to obtain different ideas that may help solve energy issues. AI can support (but not replace) technicians in decision-making. (Chatterjee & Dethlefs, 2022). Awareness of all energies can help prevent acute and chronic illnesses and energy issues raised throughout this chapter and text. This focus is possible when the scientific method impeccably derives findings and conclusions backing theories for recommended guidelines and best practices.

A magnetic (energy) field connects animal and human communication as established in human brain activity by magnetoencephalography. (Hosseini, 2021). This finding suggests the potentiality of constant telepathic communication. Two participants (Rao et al., 2014), and three human subjects (Jiang et al., 2019), demonstrated cooperation in performing tasks through this brain-brain communication. Some people experience a higher sense of self-communication as a gut feeling or intuition (the intersection of matching vibrations and frequencies). Are all aspects of life intrinsically linked to allow for communication that allows for coincidences? All living things (including unicellular organisms and plants) communicate and attempt to survive. The absence of a nervous system or nucleus may lead people to disregard their sentience. Some actions are done using electrical signals (unicellular quorum sensing) and calcium ion messenger molecules (plants) (DeFalco et al., 2023), with the same results.

Many believe the cosmic ether accounts for some of the mysterious occurrences within the natural world. Some say that the 1887 Michelson-Morley interferometer experiment was unable to produce the existence of the cosmic ether (a medium for electromagnetic waves) due to its limitations. Since then, scientists have used radio frequencies, light-beam interferometers, and other methods (Roychoudhuri, 2021), to support its existence. Thirteen points support the existence of a quantum field or ether. These points say that the "quantum field is the modern form of ether and meets the standard of being called the luminiferous ether" (Ray Fleming, 2020). Some people claim that everything exists in the ether. Then one can see that all possibilities can be transmitted and received via electromagnetic waves. They then realize that electromagnetic waves can transmit and receive all possibilities. Initially, this thought contradicted Albert Einstein's 1905 Special Theory of Relativity. In 1920 Einstein stated, "Recapitulating, we may say that according to the general theory of relativity space is endowed with physical qualities; in this sense, therefore, there exists an ether."

The debate about the unexplainable, including biogenesis, continues. How ever one believes life originated, humans can be perceived as part of that nascency. Personal perceptions of life have created problems in relationships when one finds it challenging to accept the existence of another's children. If one believes in the interconnectedness of all, they can view children as part of a shared source. An authority figure once told a child that only biological relatives *mattered. This belief alienates and demeans the existence of foster and adopted children, stepchildren, stepparents, and stepfamilies. However, human beings have binding qualities in common ancestors and in their biological makeup (99.9% of the human genome is identical). (NIH, 2017). In other words, humans consist of identical particles expressing various physical and personal characteristics. Instead of focusing on the obvious differences, one can choose to recognize commonalities, creating a feeling of connectedness to one another and other living systems, and allow others to feel their connections. A deceptive reality is created when one's truth originates from *fear, then, life can become one of illusions (Chapter 2).

People exercise power by discerning and deflecting bias, fear, and emotional spin, regardless of what others declare as fact. Then, through the all-encompassing field, the energies one chooses connects to the collective. Compassion and love translate to actions collectively contributing to humanity and the planet's energy (frequency and vibration). Some believe everyone and everything has a purpose on Earth and in the Universe. The first law of thermodynamics posits that energy is neither created nor destroyed; it changes form or is transferred from one place to another (Chapter 8). In pertaining to the human system, one can believe that we are, have always been, and will always be energy in some type of form. As energy is a universal construct affecting all living systems, people can learn to use it more efficiently. This has particular relevance when imparting the transfer of energies throughout the world. If a field unites everyone, individual and collective thoughts and prayers can transmit the energy of peace to the global population. Public officials commonly use these incarnations, which imply telepathic delivery, in their statements of compassion after tragedies. Others can only recognize peace when they realize it within themselves. "Each one has to find his peace from within. And peace, to be real, must be unaffected by outside circumstances" (Mahatma Gandi). "When the power of love overcomes the love of power, the world will know peace" (Mahatma Gandi).

Individual and global discord is transmuted when world leaders and all people realize their interconnectedness while embodying love, harmony, and peace, cultivating respect. This is the evolution of true personal power (taking control of one's own life without trying to control others). These practices promote inner peace, paving the way for world peace. Each person cultivating a sense of tranquility within contributes to a more harmonious society. "We but mirror the world. All the tendencies present in the outer world are to be found in the world of our body. If we could change ourselves, the tendencies in the world would also change" (Mahatma Gandhi). Each person choosing to consistently engage in peaceful perspectives favorably shifts unity within themselves, the world, the planet, and beyond.

# END NOTES

Reworded denotation reflects rewording to retain original content.

Listed below are the links to the creative commons licenses of articles.

This is the link address for the creative commons licenses for articles under the http://creativecommons.org/licenses/by/4.0/.

The Creative Commons Public Domain Dedication waiver (http://creativecommons.org/publicdomain/zero/1.0/).
Anyone associated with this work waivered their rights. No permission is required to use this work and there are no warranties about the work. When using or citing the work, you should not imply endorsement by the author or the affirmer. Author's note: The use of these articles does not imply endorsement of this article's contents, product, or anything else.

(http://creativecommons.org/licenses/by/2.0. Share, copy and redistribute the material in any medium or format for any purpose, even commercially. You must give appropriate credit , provide a link to the license, and indicate if changes were made_. You may do so in any reasonable manner, but not in any way that suggests the licensor endorses you or your use. Author's note: The use of these articles does not imply endorsement of this article's contents, product, or anything else.

Open Access article distributed under the terms of the Creative Commons Attribution License, (http://creativecommons.org/licenses/by/3.0/) which permits unrestricted use, distribution, and reproduction in any medium, provided the original work is properly cited.

Open-access article distributed under the terms of the Creative Commons Attribution License (CC BY). The use, distribution or reproduction in other forums is permitted, provided the original author(s) and the copyright owner(s) are credited and that the original publication in this journal is cited, in accordance with accepted academic practice.

Open-access article distributed under the terms of the Creative Commons Attribution License, which permits unrestricted use, distribution, and reproduction in any medium, provided the original work is properly cited.

Open-access articles distributed under the terms of the Creative Commons Attribution 4.0 International License (http://creativecommons.org/licenses/by/4.0/), which permits unrestricted use, distribution, and reproduction in any medium, provided you give appropriate credit to the original author(s) and the source, provide a link to the Creative Commons license, and indicate if changes were made.

Articles are licensed under a Creative Commons Attribution 4.0 International License, which permits use, sharing, adaptation, distribution and reproduction in any medium or format, as long as you give appropriate credit to the original author(s) and the source, provide a link to the Creative Commons license, and indicate if changes were made. The images or other third-party material in this article are included in the article's Creative Commons license, unless indicated otherwise in a credit line to the material. If material is not included in the article's Creative Commons license and your intended use is not permitted by statutory regulation or exceeds the permitted use, you will need to obtain permission directly from the copyright holder. To view a copy of this license, visit http://creativecommons.org/licenses/by/4.0/.

## Preface:

Di Domenico SI, Ryan RM. The Emerging Neuroscience of Intrinsic Motivation: A New Frontier in Self-Determination Research. *Front Hum Neurosci.* 2017 Mar 24;11:145. doi: 10.3389/fnhum.2017.00145. PMID: 28392765; PMCID: PMC5364176. Copyright © 2017 Di Domenico and Ryan. This is an open-access article distributed under the terms of the Creative Commons Attribution License (CC BY). Reworded.

Colloca L. The Nocebo Effect. *Annu Rev Pharmacol Toxicol.* 2024 Jan 23;64:171-190. doi: 10.1146/annurev-pharmtox-022723-112425. Epub 2023 Aug 16. PMID: 37585661; PMCID: PMC10868531. This work is licensed under a **Creative Commons Attribution 4.0 International License. Reworded.**

Arkes HR, Aberegg SK, Arpin KA. Analysis of Physicians' Probability Estimates of a Medical Outcome Based on a Sequence of Events. JAMA Netw Open. 2022 Jun 1;5(6):e2218804. doi: 10.1001/jamanetworkopen.2022.18804. PMID: 35759260; PMCID: PMC9237793. Copyright 2022 Arkes HR et al. *JAMA Network Open.* This is an open access article distributed under the terms of the CC-BY License. Quote.

Ibid, quote.

https://www.cms.gov/priorities/key-initiatives/open-payments

Teixeira da Silva JA, Dobránszki J, Bhar RH, Mehlman CT. Editors Should Declare Conflicts of Interest. J Bioeth Inq. 2019 Jun;16(2):279-298. doi: 10.1007/s11673-019-09908-2. Epub 2019 Apr 23. PMID: 31016681;

PMCID: PMC6598958. © The Author(s) 2019. Open Access This article is distributed under the terms of the Creative Commons Attribution 4.0 International License (http://creativecommons.org/licenses/by/4.0/). Reworded.

**Introduction:**

Lyons SM, Alizadeh E, Mannheimer J, Schuamberg K, Castle J, Schroder B, Turk P, Thamm D, Prasad A. Changes in cell shape are correlated with metastatic potential in murine and human osteosarcomas. *Biol Open*. 2016 Feb 12;5(3):289-99. doi: 10.1242/bio.013409. PMID: 26873952; PMCID: PMC4810736. © 2016. Published by The Company of Biologists Ltd. http://creativecommons.org/licenses/by/3.0. Reworded.

https://www.youtube.com/watch?v=yGYTLOGZ40U&ab_channel=MayoClinic. Panos Anastasadis, PH.D., (*Mayo Clinic Researchers Find New Code That Makes Reprogramming of Cancer Cells Possible*), 2015

Koury J, Lucero M, Cato C, Chang L, Geiger J, Henry D, Hernandez J, Hung F, Kaur P, Teskey G, Tran A. Immunotherapies: Exploiting the Immune System for Cancer Treatment. *J Immunol Res*. 2018 Mar 14;2018:9585614. doi: 10.1155/2018/9585614. PMID: 29725606; PMCID: PMC5872614. Copyright © 2018 Jeffrey Koury et al This is an open access article distributed under the Creative Commons Attribution License. Reworded.

https://www.congress.gov/bill/115th-congress/house-bill/2368

Baluška F, Miller WB Jr, Reber AS. Biomolecular Basis of Cellular Consciousness via Subcellular Nanobrains. *Int J Mol Sci*. 2021 Mar 3;22(5):2545. doi: 10.3390/ijms22052545. PMID: 33802617; PMCID: PMC7961929. © 2021 by the authors. Licensee MDPI, Basel, Switzerland. This article is an open access article distributed under the terms and conditions of the Creative Commons Attribution (CC BY) license. Reworded.

Rao TS, Asha MR, Jagannatha Rao KS, Vasudevaraju P. The biochemistry of belief. *Indian J Psychiatry*. 2009 Oct-Dec;51(4):239-41. doi: 10.4103/0019-5545.58285. PMID: 20048445; PMCID: PMC2802367. This is an open-access article distributed under the terms of the Creative Commons Attribution License. Quote.

Ibid, Rao et al., 2009, quote.

Ibid, Colloca, 2023, quote.

**Chapter 1: The Conundrum of Health**

https://www.nih.gov/news-events/news-releases/scientists-replay-movie-encoded-dna

*Clonal Expansion of Blood Stem Cells in Aging and Leukemia with Leonard Zon*, November 1, 2023. https://www.youtube.com/watch?v=cuVE8OpnhN4

Qian W, Yang W, Zhang Y, Bowen CR, Yang Y. Piezoelectric Materials for Controlling Electro-Chemical Processes. *Nanomicro Lett.* 2020 Jul 14;12(1):149. doi: 10.1007/s40820-020-00489-z. PMID: 34138166; PMCID: PMC7770897. © The Author(s) 2020. Open Access. This article is licensed under a Creative Commons Attribution 4.0 International License. To view a copy of this license, visit http://creativecommons.org/licenses/by/4.0/. Reworded.

Zaszczyńska A, Gradys A, Sajkiewicz P. Progress in the Applications of Smart Piezoelectric Materials for Medical Devices. *Polymers* (Basel). 2020 Nov 22;12(11):2754. doi: 10.3390/polym12112754. PMID: 33266424; PMCID: PMC7700596. © 2020 by the authors. © 2020 by the authors. Licensee MDPI, Basel, Switzerland. This article is an open access article distributed under the terms and conditions of the Creative Commons Attribution (CC BY) license (http://creativecommons.org/licenses/by/4.0/. Quote.

Kao FC, Chiu PY, Tsai TT, Lin ZH. The application of nanogenerators and piezoelectricity in osteogenesis. *Sci Technol Adv Mater.* 2019 Nov 19;20(1):1103-1117. doi: 10.1080/14686996.2019.1693880. PMID: 32002085; PMCID: PMC6968561. © 2019 The Author(s). Published by National Institute for Materials Science in partnership with Taylor & Francis Group. This is an Open Access article distributed under the terms of the Creative Commons Attribution License (http://creativecommons.org/licenses/by/4.0/. Quote.

Rao TS, Asha MR, Jagannatha Rao KS, Vasudevaraju P. The biochemistry of belief. *Indian J Psychiatry.* 2009 Oct-Dec;51(4):239-41. doi: 10.4103/0019-5545.58285. PMID: 20048445; PMCID: PMC2802367. This is an open-access article distributed under the terms of the Creative Commons Attribution License. Reworded.

*Epigenetics, Consciousness, & Reprogramming the Mind - Dr Bruce Lipton*, April 11, 2024, https://www.youtube.com/watch?v=FZexbpHLc_g

Aydin C, Kalkan R. Cancer Treatment: An Epigenetic View. *Glob Med Genet.* 2020 Jun;7(1):3-7. doi: 10.1055/s-0040-1713610. Epub 2020 Jul 15. PMID: 32879917; PMCID: PMC7410103. This is an open-access article distributed under the terms of the Creative Commons Attribution License. Reworded.

Hansen E, Zech N. Nocebo Effects and Negative Suggestions in Daily Clinical Practice - Forms, Impact and Approaches to Avoid Them. *Front Pharmacol.* 2019 Feb 13;10:77. doi: 10.3389/fphar.2019.00077. PMID: 30814949; PMCID: PMC6381056. Copyright © 2019 Hansen and Zech. This is an open-access article distributed under the terms of the Creative Commons Attribution License (CC BY). Reworded.

Ibid. Rao et al., 2009, reworded.

https://www.cdc.gov/nchs/data/nhsr/nhsr018.pdf

https://www.who.int/initiatives/who-global-centre-for-traditional-medicine

*Texas Doctor Using Right To Try Law to Treat Cancer,* Ebrahim Delpassan, MD, September 22, 2016. *Patientshttps://www.youtube.com/watch?v=JxTyHOypyac&ab_channel=Goldwater Institute.*

*Luncheon with the Experts: Ebrahim S. Delpassand, MD,* Interviewed by Rayne Bennetts, April 13, 2021 https://www.youtube.com/watch?v=4A6HN-liuq4&t=143s&ab_channel=CarcinoidCancerFoundation.

https://www.govinfo.gov/content/pkg/CHRG-114shrg22718/html/CHRG-114shrg22718.htm

https://www.congress.gov/bill/115th-congress/house-bill/2368

Health Organization. Who.int, 2017. Web 1 May 2017. Health. 2018. World Health Organization.com. Retrieved January 5, 2018, from https://www.who.int/about/who-we-are/constitution.

https://www.who.int/data/gho/data/major-themes/health-and-well-being

"Health" Merriam-Webster.com. Merriam-Webster, 2018 Web. 1 December 2018, quote.

"What affects Health" CDC.gov Centers for Disease Control, 2019. Web. 2, January 2019.

Svalastog AL, Donev D, Jahren Kristoffersen N, Gajović S. Concepts and definitions of health and health-related values in the knowledge landscapes of the digital society. *Croat Med J.* 2017 Dec 31;58(6):431-435. doi: 10.3325/cmj.2017.58.431. PMID: 29308835; PMCID: PMC5778676. Copyright © 2017 by the Croatian Medical Journal. All rights reserved. This is an open access article distributed under the Creative Commons Attribution License. Quote.

https://www.nccih.nih.gov/about/nccih-strategic-plan-2021-2025#

Ibid, www.nccih.hih,gov

Harrad R, Cosentino C, Keasley R, Sulla F. Spiritual care in nursing: an overview of the measures used to assess spiritual care provision and related factors amongst nurses. *Acta Biomed.* 2019 Mar 28;90(4-S):44-55. doi: 10.23750/abm.v90i4-S.8300. PMID: 30977748; PMCID: PMC6625560. Copyright: © 2019 ACTA BIO MEDICA SOCIETY OF MEDICINE AND NATURAL SCIENCES OF PARMA. Copyright: © 2019 ACTA BIO MEDICA SOCIETY OF MEDICINE AND NATURAL SCIENCES OF PARMA. This work is licensed under a Creative Commons Attribution 4.0 International License. Reworded.

https://www.jointcommission.org/standards/standard-faqs/critical-access-hospital/provision-of-care-treatm

## Chapter 2: Perception: Reality Versus Illusion

Moya P. Habit and embodiment in Merleau-Ponty. *Front Hum Neurosci.* 2014 Jul 25;8:542. doi: 10.3389/fnhum.2014.00542. Erratum in: Front Hum Neurosci. 2015;9:226. PMID: 25120448; PMCID: PMC4110438. Copyright © 2014 Moya. This is an open-access article distributed under the terms of the Creative Commons Attribution License (CC BY). Quote.

Rao TS, Asha MR, Jagannatha Rao KS, Vasudevaraju P. The biochemistry of belief. *Indian J Psychiatry.* 2009 Oct-Dec;51(4):239-41. doi: 10.4103/0019-5545.58285. PMID: 20048445; PMCID: PMC2802367 This is an open-access article distributed under the terms of the Creative Commons Attribution License. Quote.

Palminteri S, Lefebvre G, Kilford EJ, Blakemore SJ. Confirmation bias in human reinforcement learning: Evidence from counterfactual feedback processing. *PLoS Comput Biol.* 2017 Aug 11;13(8):e1005684. doi: 10.1371/journal.pcbi.1005684. PMID: 28800597; PMCID: PMC5568446.© 2017 Palminteri et al. © 2017 Palminteri et al. This is an open access article distributed under the terms of the Creative Commons Attribution License. Reworded.

Giacobbi PR Jr, Stewart J, Chaffee K, Jaeschke AM, Stabler M, Kelley GA. A Scoping Review of Health Outcomes Examined in Randomized Controlled Trials Using Guided Imagery. *Prog Prev Med* (N Y). 2017 Dec;2(7):e0010. doi: 10.1097/pp9.0000000000000010. PMID: 29457147; PMCID: PMC5812272.8. Copyright © 2017 The Author(s). Published by Wolters Kluwer on behalf of the European Society of Preventive Medicine. Copyright © 2017 The Author(s). Published by Wolters Kluwer on behalf of the European Society of Preventive Medicine. This is an open access article distributed under the Creative Commons Attribution License 4.0 (CCBY). Partial quote.

Carbon CC. Understanding human perception by human-made illusions. *Front Hum Neurosci*. 2014 Jul 31;8:566. doi: 10.3389/fnhum.2014.00566. PMID: 25132816; PMCID: PMC4116780. Copyright © 2014 Carbon. This is an open-access article distributed under the terms of the Creative Commons Attribution License (CC BY). Reworded.

Molins F, Martínez-Tomás C, Serrano MÁ. Implicit Negativity Bias Leads to Greater Loss Aversion and Learning during Decision-Making. Int J Environ Res Public Health. 2022 Dec 19;19(24):17037. doi: 10.3390/ijerph192417037. PMID: 36554918; PMCID: PMC9779195. Licensee MDPI, Basel, Switzerland. This article is an open access article distributed under the terms and conditions of the Creative Commons Attribution (CC BY) license. Reworded.

Bornstein AM, Khaw MW, Shohamy D, Daw ND. Reminders of past choices bias decisions for reward in humans. *Nat Commun*. 2017 Jun 27;8:15958. doi: 10.1038/ncomms15958. PMID: 28653668; PMCID: PMC5490260. Copyright © 2017, The Author(s). Open Access This article is licensed under a Creative Commons Attribution 4.0 International License. Reworded to retain original content. To view a copy of this license, visit http://creativecommons.org/licenses/by/4.0/. Reworded.

Banerjee S, Grover S, Sridharan D. Unraveling Causal Mechanisms of Top-Down and Bottom-Up Visuospatial Attention with Non-invasive Brain Stimulation. *J Indian Inst Sci*. 2019 Jun 14;97(4):451-475. doi: 10.1007/S41745-017-0046-0. Epub 2017 Dec 6. PMID: 31231154; PMCID: PMC6588534. © The Author(s) 2017. Open Access. This article is distributed under the terms of the Creative Commons Attribution 4.0 International License (http://creativecommons.org/licenses/by/4.0/. Partial quote.

Martínez-Pernía D. Experiential Neurorehabilitation: A Neurological Therapy Based on the Enactive Paradigm. Front Psychol. 2020 May 15;11:924. doi: 10.3389/fpsyg.2020.00924. PMID: 32499741; PMCID: PMC7242721. Copyright © 2020 by the author (Martínez-Pernía). Creative Commons Attribution License (CC BY). Partial quote.

A Course in Miracles, Combined Volume Third Edition, Foundation for Inner Peace: ACIM (T-21V.1-5 p 456).

Hansen E, Zech N. Nocebo Effects and Negative Suggestions in Daily Clinical Practice - Forms, Impact and Approaches to Avoid Them. *Front Pharmacol*. 2019 Feb 13;10:77. doi: 10.3389/fphar.2019.00077. PMID: 30814949; PMCID: PMC6381056. his is an open-access article distributed under the terms of the Creative Commons Attribution License (CC BY). Reworded.

A Course in Miracles Combined Volume Third Edition, Foundation for Inner Peace ACIM (Preface, p. x).

Lindahl JR, Cooper DJ, Fisher NE, Kirmayer LJ, Britton WB. Progress or Pathology? Differential Diagnosis and Intervention Criteria for Meditation-Related Challenges: Perspectives From Buddhist Meditation Teachers and Practitioners. *Front Psychol.* 2020 Jul 29;11:1905. doi: 10.3389/fpsyg.2020.01905. PMID: 32849115; PMCID: PMC7403193. Copyright © 2020 Lindahl, Cooper, Fisher, Kirmayer and Britton. This is an open-access article distributed under the terms of the Creative Commons Attribution License (CC BY). Quote.

https://www.jointcommission.org/standards/standard-faqs/critical-access-hospital/provision-of-care-treatment-and-services-pc/000001669/

A Course in Miracles, Combined Volume Third Edition, Foundation for Inner Peace: ACIM (T-30VIII.1:2 p. 643).

Subedi B, Grossberg GT. Phantom limb pain: mechanisms and treatment approaches. *Pain Res Treat.* 2011;2011:864605. doi: 10.1155/2011/864605. Epub 2011 Aug 14. PMID: 22110933; PMCID: PMC3198614. Copyright © 2011 B. Subedi and G. T. Grossberg. open access article distributed under the Creative Commons Attribution License. Quote.

A Course in Miracles, Combined Volume Third Edition, Foundation for Inner Peace ACIM (T-21V.1 p. 456).

A Course in Miracles, Combined Volume Third Edition, Foundation for Inner Peace ACIM (T-21V.2 p. 456).

*Man With 'Walking Corpse Syndrome' Thought He Was* Dead, Good Morning Britain 2/12/16
https://www.youtube.com/watch?v=7k7ckxjrRqM&ab_channel=Good MorningBritain

Varieties of perceptual instability and their neural correlates Tomohiro Ishizu, Semir Zeki *Neuroimage.* 2014 May 1; 91(100): 203–209. doi: 10.1016/j.neuroimage.2014.01.040 PMCID: PMC3985424. © 2014 The Authors This is an open-access article distributed under the terms of the Creative Commons Attribution License. Reworded.

Ishizu T. Disambiguation of ambiguous figures in the brain. *Front Hum Neurosci.* 2013 Aug 30;7:501. doi: 10.3389/fnhum.2013.00501. PMID: 24009570; PMCID: PMC3757299. Commons Attribution License (CC BY). Reworded.

Ibid, Ishizu, 2013, quote.

https://science.nasa.gov/solar-system/moon/the-moon-illusion-why-does-the-moon-look-so-big-sometimes/

Ibid, Hansen & Zech, 2019, reworded.

A Course in Miracles Combined Volume Third Edition, Foundation for Inner Peace Preface, p. x.

A Course in Miracles Combined Volume Third Edition Foundation for Inner Peace ACIM (T-3.111.8 p. 40).

Rao TS, Asha MR, Jagannatha Rao KS, Vasudevaraju P. The biochemistry of belief. *Indian J Psychiatry*. 2009 Oct-Dec;51(4):239-41. doi: 10.4103/0019-5545.58285. PMID: 20048445; PMCID: PMC2802367. © Indian Journal of Psychiatry. This is an open-access article distributed under the terms of the Creative Commons Attribution License. Quote.

Van Hoeck N, Watson PD, Barbey AK. Cognitive neuroscience of human counterfactual reasoning. *Front Hum Neurosci*. 2015 Jul 23;9:420. doi: 10.3389/fnhum.2015.00420. PMID: 26257633; PMCID: PMC4511878. Copyright © 2015 Van Hoeck, Watson and Barbey. This is an open-access article distributed under the terms of the Creative Commons Attribution License (CC BY). Reworded.

Clark IA, Mackay CE. Mental Imagery and Post-Traumatic Stress Disorder: A Neuroimaging and Experimental Psychopathology Approach to Intrusive Memories of Trauma. *Front Psychiatry*. 2015 Jul 22;6:104. doi: 10.3389/fpsyt.2015.00104. PMID: 26257660; PMCID: PMC4510312. Copyright © 2015 Clark and Mackay. This is an open-access article distributed under the terms of the Creative Commons Attribution License (CC BY). Reworded.

Ramsey LA, Koya E, van den Oever MC. Editorial: Neuronal ensembles and memory engrams: Cellular and molecular mechanisms. *Front Behav Neurosci*. 2023 Feb 28;17:1157414. doi: 10.3389/fnbeh.2023.1157414. PMID: 36926583; PMCID: PMC10011704. Copyright © 2023 Ramsey, Koya and van den Oever. This is an open-access article distributed under the terms of the Creative Commons Attribution License (CC BY). Reworded.

Iqbal J, Huang GD, Xue YX, Yang M, Jia XJ. The neural circuits and molecular mechanisms underlying fear dysregulation in posttraumatic stress disorder. *Front Neurosci*. 2023 Dec 5;17:1281401. doi: 10.3389/fnins.2023.1281401. PMID: 38116070; PMCID: PMC10728304.Copyright © 2023 Iqbal, Huang, Xue, Yang and Jia. This is an open-access article distributed under the terms of the Creative Commons Attribution License (CC BY). Reworded.

*CYMATICS: Science Vs. Music* - Nigel Stanford 1 Hour, August 1 2021 https://www.youtube.com/watch?v=Ace2da4TFz4&ab_channel=SJBeat s

*Gregg Braden, Bladder Cancer dissolves in less than 3 minutes using The Language of Emotion,* Gregg Braydon 2011, https://www.youtube.com/watch?v=GUbEgg6GklU&ab_channel=Worl dClassWellness

Serafini B, Rosicarelli B, Veroni C, Mazzola GA, Aloisi F. Epstein-Barr Virus-Specific CD8 T Cells Selectively Infiltrate the Brain in Multiple Sclerosis and Interact Locally with Virus-Infected Cells: Clue for a Virus-Driven Immunopathological Mechanism. *J Virol.* 2019 Nov 26;93(24):e00980-19. doi: 10.1128/JVI.00980-19. PMID: 31578295; PMCID: PMC6880158. Copyright © 2019 Serafini et al. Creative Commons Attribution 4.0 International license. Reworded.

**Chapter 3: The Scope and Efficacy of Scientific Research.**

Di Domenico SI, Ryan RM. The Emerging Neuroscience of Intrinsic Motivation: A New Frontier in Self-Determination Research. *Front Hum Neurosci.* 2017 Mar 24;11:145. doi: 10.3389/fnhum.2017.00145. PMID: 28392765; PMCID: PMC5364176. Copyright © 2017 Di Domenico and Ryan. This is an open-access article distributed under the terms of the Creative Commons Attribution License (CC BY). Reworded.

Mousavi S. Global Ethical Principles in Healthcare Networks, Including Debates on Euthanasia and Abortion. *Cureus.* 2024 Apr 26;16(4):e59116. doi: 10.7759/cureus.59116. PMID: 38803720; PMCID: PMC11128767. Copyright © 2024, Mousavi et al. This is an open access article distributed under the terms of the Creative Commons Attribution License CC-BY 4.0. Quote.

Olsson TM, Sundell K. Publication bias, time-lag bias, and place-of-publication bias in social intervention research: An exploratory study of 527 Swedish articles published between 1990-2019. *PLoS One.* 2023 Feb 6;18(2):e0281110. doi: 10.1371/journal.pone.0281110. PMID: 36745625; PMCID: PMC9901762. © 2023 Olsson, Sundell. This is an open access article distributed under the terms of the Creative Commons Attribution License. Reworded.

Ross PT, Bibler Zaidi NL. Limited by our limitations. *Perspect Med Educ.* 2019 Aug;8(4):261-264. doi: 10.1007/s40037-019-00530-x. PMID: 31347033; PMCID: PMC6684501. © The Author(s) 2019. © The Author(s) 2019. Open Access. This article is distributed under the terms of the

Creative Commons Attribution 4.0 International License (http://creativecommons.org/licenses/by/4.0/. Reworded.

Herrera-Perez D, Haslam A, Crain T, Gill J, Livingston C, Kaestner V, Hayes M, Morgan D, Cifu AS, Prasad V. A comprehensive review of randomized clinical trials in three medical journals reveals 396 medical reversals. *Elife*. 2019 Jun 11;8:e45183. doi: 10.7554/eLife.45183. PMID: 31182188; PMCID: PMC6559784. © 2019, Herrera-Perez et al. This article is distributed under the terms of the Creative Commons Attribution License. Reworded.

Herrera-Perez et al., 2019, ibid, reworded.

https://www.nih.gov/news-events/nih-research-matters/aspirin-use-may-be-widespread-despite-new-guidelines

Luo H, Ge H. Hot Tea Consumption and Esophageal Cancer Risk: A Meta-Analysis of Observational Studies. *Front Nutr*. 2022 Apr 11;9:831567. doi: 10.3389/fnut.2022.831567. PMID: 35479756; PMCID: PMC9035825. Copyright © 2022 Luo and Ge. This is an open-access article distributed under the terms of the Creative Commons Attribution License (CC BY). Reworded.

Ioannidis JP. Why most published research findings are false. *PLoS Med*. 2005;2(8):e124. doi:10.1371/journal.pmed.0020124. Copyright: © 2005 John P. A. Ioannidis. This is an open-access article distributed under the terms of the Creative Commons Attribution License. Quote.

https://oceanservice.noaa.gov/facts/earth-round.html

TEDx Talks. (2012, October 1). *The Half-Life of Facts: Sam Arbesman at TEDxKC* (Video) YouTube. *https://www.youtube.com/watch?v=GaxYnvd7YAM&ab_channel=TEDxTalks*

Jozi Z, Nourmohammadi H. Scientometrics Analysis of World Scientific Research of Pathology and Forensic Medicine. *Iran J Pathol*. 2022 Spring;17(2):191-201. doi: 10.30699/ijp.2022.541660.2756. Epub 2022 Feb 20. PMID: 35463726; PMCID: PMC9013873. This is an Open Access article distributed under the terms of the Creative Commons Attribution License, (http://creativecommons.org/licenses/by/3.0/ Reworded.

Ibid, Jozi & Nourmohammadi, 2022, reworded.

Jonas WB, Crawford C, Hilton L, Elfenbaum P. Scientific Evaluation and Review of Claims in Health Care (SEaRCH): A Streamlined, Systematic, Phased Approach for Determining "What Works" in Healthcare. *J Altern Complement Med*. 2017 Jan;23(1):18-25. doi: 10.1089/acm.2016.0291. Epub

2016 Dec 27. PMID: 28026968; PMCID: PMC5248545. This is an Open Access article distributed under the terms of the Creative Commons Attribution License, (http://creativecommons.org/licenses/by/3.0/ Reworded.

Chong MC, Sharp MK, Smith SM, O'Neill M, Ryan M, Lynch R, Mahtani KR, Clyne B. Strong recommendations from low certainty evidence: a cross-sectional analysis of a suite of national guidelines. *BMC Med Res Methodol.* 2023 Mar 25;23(1):68. doi: 10.1186/s12874-023-01895-8. PMID: 36966277; PMCID: PMC10039768. © The Author(s) 2023. CC 4.0. https://creativecommons.org/publicdomain/zero/1.0/. The use of this article cited within this article does not imply endorsement of any article contents, product, or anything else. Reworded.

The answer is 17 years, what is the question: understanding time lags in translational research. Zoë Slote Morris, Steven Wooding, Jonathan Grant *J R Soc Med.* 2011 Dec; 104(12): 510–520. doi: 10.1258/jrsm.2011.110180 PMCID: PMC324151 © 2011 The Royal Society of Medicine. © 2011 The Royal Society of Medicine. This is an open-access article distributed under the terms of the Creative Commons Attribution License. Reworded.

Ibid, Morris et al., 2011, reworded.

Moving Beyond Traditional Null Hypothesis Testing: Evaluation Expectations Directly. *Frontiers of Psychology* Rens Van de Schoot, Herbert Hoijtink, Romeijn Jan-WillemFront Psychol. 2011; 2: 24. Published online 2011 Feb 22. doi: 10.3389/fpsyg.2011.00024 PMCID: PMC3111216. Van de Schoot, Hoijtink and Jan-Willem. Copyright © 2011 Van de Schoot, Hoijtink and Jan-Willem. This is an open-access article subject to an exclusive license agreement between the authors and Frontiers Media SA, which permits unrestricted use, distribution, and reproduction in any medium, provided the original authors and source are credited. Quote.

Banerjee A, Chitnis UB, Jadhav SL, Bhawalkar JS, Chaudhury S. Hypothesis testing, type I and type II errors. *Ind Psychiatry J.* 2009 Jul;18(2):127-31. doi: 10.4103/0972-6748.62274. PMID: 21180491; PMCID: PMC2996198. © Industrial Psychiatry Journal. This is an open-access article distributed under the terms of the Creative Commons Attribution License. Quote.

Kumar S, Chong I. Correlation Analysis to Identify the Effective Data in Machine Learning: Prediction of Depressive Disorder and Emotion States. *Int J Environ Res Public Health.* 2018 Dec 19;15(12):2907. doi: 10.3390/ijerph15122907. PMID: 30572595; PMCID: PMC6313491. © 2018 by the authors. © 2018 by the authors. Licensee MDPI, Basel, Switzerland. This article is an open access article distributed under the terms and conditions of the Creative Commons Attribution (CC BY) license (http://creativecommons.org/licenses/by/4.0/. Reworded.

Lytsy P, Hartman M, Pingel R. Misinterpretations of P-values and statistical tests persists among researchers and professionals working with statistics and epidemiology. *Ups J Med Sci.* 2022 Aug 4;127. doi: 10.48101/ujms.v127.8760. PMID: 35991465; PMCID: PMC9383044. © 2022 The Author(s). Published by Upsala Medical Society. © 2022 The Author(s). Published by Upsala Medical Society. This is an Open Access article distributed under the terms of the Creative Commons Attribution License. Quote.

Ibid, Ross & Bibler Zaidi, 2019, quote.

Open Science Collaboration. (2015). Estimating the reproducibility of psychological science. *Science, 349*(6251), aac4716. Doi: 10.1126/science.aac4716.

Wu KS, Lee SS, Chen JK, Chen YS, Tsai HC, Chen YJ, Huang YH, Lin HS. Identifying heterogeneity in the Hawthorne effect on hand hygiene observation: a cohort study of overtly and covertly observed results. *BMC Infect Dis.* 2018 Aug 6;18(1):369. doi: 10.1186/s12879-018-3292-5. PMID: 30081843; PMCID: PMC6090841. © The Author(s). 2018. Open Access. This article is distributed under the terms of the Creative Commons Attribution 4.0 International License (http://creativecommons.org/licenses/by/4.0/). The Creative Commons Public Domain Dedication waiver (http://creativecommons.org/publicdomain/zero/1.0/. Reworded. The use of this article does not imply endorsement of this article's contents, product, or anything else. Reworded.

https://osf.io

osf.io/ud578

https://osf.io/2sk9f

Evan Mayo-Wilson, E., Grant, S., Supplee, L. *et al.* Evaluating implementation of the Transparency and Openness Promotion (TOP) guidelines: the TRUST process for rating journal policies, procedures, and practices. *Res Integr Peer Rev* 6, 9 (2021). https://doi.org/10.1186/s41073-021-0011 Complete author names of this paper: Evan Mayo-Wilson, Sean Grant, Lauren Supplee, Sina Kianersi, Afsah Amin, Alex DeHaven & David Mellor Received22 January 2021 Accepted07 May 2021 Published02 June 2021 DOIhttps://doi.org/10.1186/s41073-021-00112-8http://creativecommons.org/licenses/by/4.0/. The Creative Commons Public Domain Dedication waiver (http://creativecommons.org/publicdomain/zero/1.0/) applies to the data made available in this article, unless otherwise stated in a credit line to the data. The use of this article does not imply endorsement of this article's contents, product, or anything else. Reworded.

Ibid, reworded.

https://osf.io/2sk9f/

Gopal AD, Wallach JD, Aminawung JA, Gonsalves G, Dal-Ré R, Miller JE, Ross JS. Adherence to the International Committee of Medical Journal Editors' (ICMJE) prospective registration policy and implications for outcome integrity: a cross-sectional analysis of trials published in high-impact specialty society journals. *Trials*. 2018 Aug 23;19(1):448. doi: 10.1186/s13063-018-2825-y. PMID: 30134950; PMCID: PMC6106722. © The Author(s). 2018. (http://creativecommons.org/publicdomain/zero/1.0/). The use of this article does not imply endorsement of this article's contents, product, or anything else. Reworded.

Sukhera J, Wodzinski M, Rehman M, Gonzalez CM. The Implicit Association Test in health professions education: A meta-narrative review. *Perspect Med Educ*. 2019;8(5):267-275. doi:10.1007/s40037-019-00533-8. © The Author(s) 2019. © The Author(s) 2019. Open Access. This article is distributed under the terms of the Creative Commons Attribution 4.0 International License (http://creativecommons.org/licenses/by/4.0/. Quote.

Openpaymentsdata.cms.gov

Averitt AJ, Weng C, Ryan P, Perotte A. Translating evidence into practice: eligibility criteria fail to eliminate clinically significant differences between real-world and study populations. *NPJ Digit Med*. 2020 May 11;3:67. doi: 10.1038/s41746-020-0277-8. PMID: 32411828; PMCID: PMC7214444. © The Author(s) 2020. Open Access This article is licensed under a Creative Commons Attribution 4.0 International License. To view a copy of this license, visit http://creativecommons.org/licenses/by/4.0/. Reworded.

Regnault A, Willgoss T, Barbic S; International Society for Quality of Life Research (ISOQOL) Mixed Methods Special Interest Group (SIG). Towards the use of mixed methods inquiry as best practice in health outcomes research. *J Patient Rep Outcomes*. 2017;2(1):19. doi: 10.1186/s41687-018-0043-8. Epub 2018 Apr 11. PMID: 29757311; PMCID: PMC5934918. © The Author(s) 2018. Open Access. This article is distributed under the terms of the Creative Commons Attribution 4.0 International License (http://creativecommons.org/licenses/by/4.0. Reworded.

WWW.precis-2.org

www.consort-statement.org

Vandenbroucke JP, von Elm E, Altman DG, Gøtzsche PC, Mulrow CD, Pocock SJ, Poole C, Schlesselman JJ, Egger M; STROBE Initiative. Strengthening the Reporting of Observational Studies in Epidemiology (STROBE): explanation and elaboration. *PLoS Med.* 2007 Oct 16;4(10):e297. doi: 10.1371/journal.pmed.0040297. PMID: 17941715; PMCID: PMC2020496. © 2007 Vandenbroucke et al. This is an open-access article distributed under the terms of the Creative Commons Attribution License. Reworded.

https://public.csr.nih.gov/AboutCSR/Address-Bias-in-Peer-Review

Regnault et al, 2017, ibid, reworded.

https://public.csr.nih.gov/AboutCSR/Address-Bias-in-Peer-Review

Murray R, Sharp M, Razidan A, Hibbitts B, Ryan M, Mahtani K, Lynch R, Smith S, O'Neill M, Schünemann H, Alonso-Coello P, Munn Z, Clyne B. Investigating how the GRADE Evidence to Decision (EtD) framework is used in Clinical Guidelines: a scoping review protocol. HRB Open Res. 2023 Sep 13;6:50. doi: 10.12688/hrbopenres.13757.1. PMID: 38779426; PMCID: PMC11109711. Copyright: © 2023 Murray R et al. Copyright: © 2023 Murray R et al. This is an open access article distributed under the terms of the Creative Commons Attribution License. Partial quote.

Shaheen N, Shaheen A, Ramadan A, Hefnawy MT, Ramadan A, Ibrahim IA, Hassanein ME, Ashour ME, Flouty O. Appraising systematic reviews: a comprehensive guide to ensuring validity and reliability. *Front Res Metr Anal.* 2023 Dec 21;8:1268045. doi: 10.3389/frma.2023.1268045. PMID: 38179256; PMCID: PMC10764628. Copyright © 2023 Shaheen, Shaheen, Ramadan, Hefnawy, Ramadan, Ibrahim, Hassanein, Ashour and Flouty. Copyright © 2023 Shaheen, Shaheen, Ramadan, Hefnawy, Ramadan, Ibrahim, Hassanein, Ashour and Flouty. This is an open-access article distributed under the terms of the Creative Commons Attribution License (CC BY). Reworded.

Mickenautsch S. Systematic reviews, systematic error and the acquisition of clinical knowledge. *BMC Med Res Methodol.* 2010 Jun 10;10:53. doi: 10.1186/1471-2288-10-53. PMID: 20537172; PMCID: PMC2897793. Copyright ©2010 Mickenautsch; licensee BioMed Central Ltd. This is an Open Access article distributed under the terms of the Creative Commons Attribution License (http://creativecommons.org/licenses/by/2.0. The use of this article does not imply endorsement of this article's contents, product, or anything else. Reworded.

Peters MDJ, Marnie C, Colquhoun H, Garritty CM, Hempel S, Horsley T, Langlois EV, Lillie E, O'Brien KK, Tunçalp Ö, Wilson MG, Zarin W, Tricco AC. Scoping reviews: reinforcing and advancing the methodology and application. *Syst Rev.* 2021 Oct 8;10(1):263. doi: 10.1186/s13643-021-01821-3. PMID: 34625095; PMCID: PMC8499488. © The Author(s) 2021. CC 4.0 and https://creativecommons.org/publicdomain/zero/1.0/. The use of this article does not imply endorsement of this article's contents, product, or anything else. Reworded.

Edelman A, Clay-Williams R, Fischer M, Kislov R, Kitson A, McLoughlin I, Skouteris H, Harvey G. Academic Health Science Centres as Vehicles for Knowledge Mobilisation in Australia? A Qualitative Study. *Int J Health Policy Manag.* 2022 Jun 1;11(6):840-846. doi: 10.34172/ijhpm.2020.247. PMID: 33590737; PMCID: PMC9309908. © 2022 The Author(s); Published by Kerman University of Medical Sciences. © 2022 The Author(s); Published by Kerman University of Medical Sciences. This is an open-access article distributed under the terms of the Creative Commons Attribution License (http://creativecommons.org/licenses/by/4.0. Reworded.

Wende ME, Wilcox S, Rhodes Z, Kinnard D, Turner-McGrievy G, McKeever BW, Kaczynski AT. Developing criteria for research translation decision-making in community settings: a systematic review and thematic analysis informed by the Knowledge to Action Framework and community input. *Implement Sci Commun.* 2022 Jul 16;3(1):76. doi: 10.1186/s43058-022-00316-z. PMID: 35850778; PMCID: PMC9290208. © The Author(s) 2022. Open Access. This article is licensed under a Creative Commons Attribution 4.0 International License. To view a copy of this licence, visit http://creativecommons.org/licenses/by/4.0/. The Creative Commons Public Domain Dedication waiver (http://creativecommons.org/publicdomain/zero/1.0/. The use of this article does not imply endorsement of this article's contents, product, or anything else. Reworded.

Huang W, Percie du Sert N, Vollert J, Rice ASC. General Principles of Preclinical Study Design. *Handb Exp Pharmacol.* 2020;257:55-69. doi: 10.1007/164_2019_277. PMID: 31707471; PMCID: PMC7610693. This chapter is licensed under the terms of the Creative Commons Attribution 4.0 International License (https://creativecommons.org/licenses/by/4.0 Partial quote.

https://www.hhs.gov/ohrp/international/compilation-human-research-standards

https://www.unesco.org/en/legal-affairs/recommendation-science-and-scientific-researchers

https://www.nal.usda.gov/animal-health-and-welfare/animal-welfare-act

https://ori.hhs.gov/association-assessment-and-accreditation-laboratory-animal-care-international-aaalac

Akhtar A. The flaws and human harms of animal experimentation. *Camb Q Healthc Ethics*. 2015 Oct;24(4):407-19. doi: 10.1017/S0963180115000079. PMID: 26364776; PMCID: PMC4594046. © Cambridge University Press 2015. This is an Open Access article, distributed under the terms of the Creative Commons Attribution license (http://creativecommons.org/licenses/by/3.0/. Reworded.

Yang Y, Litscher G, Sun Z, Sun W. The Application of Laser Acupuncture in Animal Experiments: A Narrative Review of Biological Aspects. *Evid Based Complement Alternat Med*. 2021 Feb 24;2021:6646237. doi: 10.1155/2021/6646237. PMID: 33680056; PMCID: PMC7929682. Copyright © 2021 Yan Yang et al. opyright © 2021 Yan Yang et al. This is an open access article distributed under the Creative Commons Attribution License. Reworded.

Domínguez-Oliva A, Hernández-Ávalos I, Martínez-Burnes J, Olmos-Hernández A, Verduzco-Mendoza A, Mota-Rojas D. The Importance of Animal Models in Biomedical Research: Current Insights and Applications. Animals (Basel). 2023 Mar 31;13(7):1223. doi: 10.3390/ani13071223. PMID: 37048478; PMCID: PMC10093480. © 2023 by the authors. Attribution (CC BY) license (https://creativecommons.org/licenses/by/4.0/. Reworded.

**Chapter 4: Overcoming Workplace Challenges**

American Nurses Association www.nursingworld.org/

practice-policy/advocacy/state/workplace-violence2/

American Nurses Association https://www.nursingworld.org/ practice-policy/ work-environment/violence-incivility-bullying/

https://www.nursingworld.org/practice-policy/advocacy/state/workplace-violence2/

https://www.ama-assn.org/press-center/press-releases/ama-adopts-new-policy-aimed-preventing-bullying-medicine

https://www.osha.gov/workplace-violence

https://www.jointcommission.org/-/media/tjc/documents/standards/r3-reports/wpvp-r3_20210618.pdf

Leach LS, Too LS, Batterham PJ, Kiely KM, Christensen H, Butterworth P. Workplace Bullying and Suicidal Ideation: Findings from an Australian Longitudinal Cohort Study of Mid-Aged Workers. *Int J Environ Res Public Health*. 2020 Feb 24;17(4):1448. doi: 10.3390/ijerph17041448. PMID: 32102336; PMCID: PMC7068571 © 2020 by the authors. Licensee MDPI, Basel, Switzerland. This article is an open access article distributed under the terms and conditions of the Creative Commons Attribution (CC BY) license (http://creativecommons.org/licenses/by/4.0/. Reworded.

https://www.nahcacna.org

https://www.nimh.nih.gov/research/research-funded-by-nimh/rdoc/constructs/circadian-rhythms

Wong K, Chan AHS, Ngan SC. The Effect of Long Working Hours and Overtime on Occupational Health: A Meta-Analysis of Evidence from 1998 to 2018. *Int J Environ Res Public Health*. 2019 Jun 13;16(12):2102. doi: 10.3390/ijerph16122102. PMID: 31200573; PMCID: PMC6617405. © 2019 by the authors. Licensee MDPI, Basel, Switzerland. This article is an open access article distributed under the terms and conditions of the Creative Commons Attribution (CC BY) license (http://creativecommons.org/licenses/by/4.0. Reworded.

Desai D, Momin A, Hirpara P, Jha H, Thaker R, Patel J. Exploring the Role of Circadian Rhythms in Sleep and Recovery: A Review Article. *Cureus*. 2024 Jun 3;16(6):e61568. doi: 10.7759/cureus.61568. PMID: 38962617; PMCID: PMC11221196. Copyright © 2024, Desai et al. This is an open access article distributed under the terms of the Creative Commons Attribution License CC-BY 4.0. Reworded.

Tran HT, Kondo T, Ashry A, Fu Y, Okawa H, Sawangmake C, Egusa H. Effect of circadian clock disruption on type 2 diabetes. *Front Physiol*. 2024 Aug 6;15:1435848. doi: 10.3389/fphys.2024.1435848. PMID: 39165284; PMCID: PMC11333352. Copyright © 2024 Tran, Kondo, Ashry, Fu, Okawa, Sawangmake and Egusa. This is an open-access article distributed under the terms of the Creative Commons Attribution License (CC BY) 4.0 Reworded.

Yaribeygi H, Panahi Y, Sahraei H, Johnston TP, Sahebkar A. The impact of stress on body function: A review. *EXCLI J*. 2017 Jul 21;16:1057-1072. doi: 10.17179/excli2017-480. PMID: 28900385; PMCID: PMC5579396. Copyright © 2017 Yaribeygi et al. Copyright © 2017 Yaribeygi et al. This is an Open Access article distributed under the terms of the Creative Commons Attribution License (http://creativecommons.org/licenses/by/4.0/. Reworded.

Adamsson A, Bernhardsson S. Symptoms that may be stress-related and lead to exhaustion disorder: a retrospective medical chart review in Swedish primary care. *BMC Fam Pract*. 2018 Oct 30;19(1):172. doi: 10.1186/s12875-018-0858-7. PMID: 30376811; PMCID: PMC6208049. © The Author(s). 2018. CC 4.0. (http://creativecommons.org/publicdomain/zero/1.0/) Reworded. The use of this article does not imply endorsement of this article's contents, product, or anything else. Reworded.

Edú-Valsania S, Laguía A, Moriano JA. Burnout: A Review of Theory and Measurement. Int *J Environ Res Public Health*. 2022 Feb 4;19(3):1780. doi: 10.3390/ijerph19031780. PMID: 35162802; PMCID: PMC8834764. © 2022 by the authors. Licensee MDPI, Basel, Switzerland. This article is an open access article distributed under the terms and conditions of the Creative Commons Attribution (CC BY) license (https://creativecommons.org/licenses/by/4.0/. Reworded.

The Shutdown Dissociation Scale (Shut-D) Inga Schalinski, Maggie Schauer, Thomas Elbert *Eur JPsychotraumatol*. 2015; 6: 10.3402/ejpt.v6.25652. Published online 2015 May 13. doi: 10.3402/ejpt.v6.25652PMCID: PMC4431999. © 2015 Inga Schalinski et al. © 2015 Inga Schalinski et al. This is an Open Access article distributed under the terms of the Creative Commons Attribution 4.0 International License. Reworded.

Ibid, Adamsson et al., 2018, reworded.

Ibid, Yaribeygi et al., 2017, reworded.

Godoy LD, Rossignoli MT, Delfino-Pereira P, Garcia-Cairasco N, de Lima Umeoka EH. A Comprehensive Overview on Stress Neurobiology: Basic Concepts and Clinical Implications. *Front Behav Neurosci*. 2018 Jul 3;12:127. doi: 10.3389/fnbeh.2018.00127. PMID: 30034327; PMCID: Copyright © 2018 Godoy, Rossignoli, Delfino-Pereira, Garcia-Cairasco and Umeoka. This is an open-access article distributed under the terms of the Creative Commons Attribution License (CC BY) CC 4.0. *

Ibid, Schalinski et al., 2015, quote.

www.nami.org

https://www.cdc.gov/nceh/radiation/ionizing_radiation.html

https://www.osha.gov/ionizing-radiation/control-prevention

Cao CF, Ma KL, Shan H, Liu TF, Zhao SQ, Wan Y, Jun-Zhang, Wang HQ. CT Scans and Cancer Risks: A Systematic Review and Dose-response Meta-analysis. *BMC Cancer*. 2022 Nov 30;22(1):1238. doi: 10.1186/s12885-022-10310-2. PMID: 36451138; PMCID: PMC9710150. © The Author(s) 2022. (http://creativecommons.org/publicdomain/zero/1.0/). The use of this article does not imply endorsement of this article's contents, product, or anything else. Reworded.

https://www.epa.gov/radiation/calculate-your-radiation-dose

Ibid, www.epa.gov

Jagetia GC. Radioprotective Potential of Plants and Herbs against the Effects of Ionizing Radiation. *J Clin Biochem Nutr*. 2007 Mar;40(2):74-81. doi: 10.3164/jcbn.40.74. PMID: 18188408; PMCID: PMC2127223. Copyright © 2007 JCBN. This is an open access article distributed under the terms of the Creative Commons Attribution License. Reworded.

https://www.cdc.gov/niosh/npg/firstaid.html

https://www.cdc.gov/niosh/topics/ergonomics/nlecalc.html

https://www.osha.gov/etools/computer-workstations

https://www.cdc.gov/niosh/topics/ergonomics/nlecalc.html

Li Y, Su Z, Li P, et al. Association of Symptoms with Eating Habits and Food Preferences in Chronic Gastritis Patients: A Cross-Sectional Study. *Evid Based Complement Alternat Med*. 2020;2020:5197201. Published 2020 Jul 9. doi:10.1155/2020/5197201. Copyright © 2020 Yuan Li et al. This is an open access article distributed under the Creative Commons Attribution License. Reworded.

Ibid, Li et al., 2020, reworded.

https://www.cdc.gov/niosh/topics/ergonomics/nlecalc.html

**Chapter 5: Patient Perspectives of Healthcare Delivery**

Smagula SF, Aizenstein HJ. Initial evidence regarding the neurobiological basis of psychological symptoms in dementia caregivers. *Transl Psychiatry*. 2023 May 18;13(1):169. doi: 10.1038/s41398-023-02457-8. PMID: 37202392; PMCID: PMC10195778. © The Author(s) 2023. Open Access. This article is licensed under a Creative Commons Attribution 4.0 International License. To view a copy of this license, visit http://creativecommons.org/licenses/by/4.0. Reworded.

Brodhun C, Borelli E, Weiss T. Neural correlates of word processing influenced by painful primes. *PLoS One*. 2024 Jan 19;19(1):e0295148. doi: 10.1371/journal.pone.0295148. PMID: 38241212; PMCID: PMC10798507. © 2024 Brodhun et al. This is an open access article distributed under the terms of the Creative Commons Attribution License. Reworded.

Matos LC, Machado JP, Monteiro FJ, Greten HJ. Perspectives, Measurability and Effects of Non-Contact Biofield-Based Practices: A Narrative Review of Quantitative Research. *Int J Environ Res Public Health*. 2021 Jun 13;18(12):6397. doi: 10.3390/ijerph18126397. PMID: 34199174; PMCID: PMC8296239. © 2021 by the authors. © 2021 by the authors. Licensee MDPI, Basel, Switzerland. This article is an open access article distributed under the terms and conditions of the Creative Commons Attribution (CC BY) license (https://creativecommons.org/licenses/by/4.0. Reworded.

Ortega Á, Salazar J, Galban N, Rojas M, Ariza D, Chávez-Castillo M, Nava M, Riaño-Garzón ME, Díaz-Camargo EA, Medina-Ortiz O, Bermúdez V. Psycho-Neuro-Endocrine-Immunological Basis of the Placebo Effect: Potential Applications beyond Pain Therapy. *Int J Mol Sci*. 2022 Apr 11;23(8):4196. doi: 10.3390/ijms23084196. PMID: 35457014; PMCID: PMC9028312. © 2022 by the authors. Licensee MDPI, Basel, Switzerland. This article is an open access article distributed under the terms and conditions of the Creative Commons Attribution (CC BY) license (https://creativecommons.org/licenses/by/4.0. Quote.

Beauvais F. Possible contribution of quantum-like correlations to the placebo effect: consequences on blind trials. *Theor Biol Med Model*. 2017 Jun 2;14(1):12. doi: 10.1186/s12976-017-0058-5. PMID: 28578662; PMCID: PMC5457621. © The Author(s). 2017 CC 4.0. The Creative Commons Public Domain Dedication waiver (http://creativecommons.org/publicdomain/zero/1.0/) applies to the data made available in this article, unless otherwise stated. The use of this article does not imply endorsement of this article's contents, product, or anything else. Quote.

Waweru E, Smekens T, Orne-Gliemann J, Ssengooba F, Broerse J, Criel B. Patient perspectives on interpersonal aspects of healthcare and patient-centeredness at primary health facilities: A mixed methods study in rural Eastern Uganda. *PLoS One*. 2020 Jul 30;15(7):e0236524. doi: 10.1371/journal.pone.0236524. PMID: 32730294; PMCID: PMC7392339. © 2020 Waweru et al. This is an open access article distributed under the terms of the Creative Commons Attribution License. Reworded.

https://www.improvediagnosis.org

https://www.jointcommission.org/standards/standard-faqs/hospital-and-hospital-clinics

Mousavi S. Global Ethical Principles in Healthcare Networks, Including Debates on Euthanasia and Abortion. Cureus. 2024 Apr 26;16(4):e59116. doi: 10.7759/cureus.59116. PMID: 38803720; PMCID: PMC11128767. Copyright © 2024, Mousavi et al. This is an open access article distributed under the terms of the Creative Commons Attribution License CC-BY 4.0. Quote.

Baluška F, Miller WB Jr, Reber AS. Biomolecular Basis of Cellular Consciousness via Subcellular Nanobrains. Int J Mol Sci. 2021 Mar

3;22(5):2545. doi: 10.3390/ijms22052545. PMID: 33802617; PMCID: PMC7961929. © 2021 by the authors. Licensee MDPI, Basel, Switzerland. This article is an open access article distributed under the terms and conditions of the Creative Commons Attribution (CC BY) license (http://creativecommons.org/licenses/by/4.0/. Reworded.

Ghaderi A, Tabatabaei SM, Nedjat S, Javadi M, Larijani B. Explanatory definition of the concept of spiritual health: a qualitative study in Iran. J Med Ethics Hist Med. 2018 Apr 9;11:3. PMID: 30258553; PMCID: PMC6150917. © 2018 Medical Ethics and History of Medicine Research Center, Tehran University of Medical Sciences. This article is distributed under the terms of the Creative Commons Attribution License, (http://creativecommons.org/licenses/by/3.0/. Reworded.

Van Bael K, Ball M, Scarfo J, Suleyman E. Assessment of the mind-body connection: preliminary psychometric evidence for a new self-report questionnaire. BMC Psychol. 2023 Oct 6;11(1):309. doi: 10.1186/s40359-023-01302-3. PMID: 37803484; PMCID: PMC10557351. © The Author(s) 2023 CC 4.0. (http://creativecommons.org/publicdomain/zero/1.0/. The use of this article does not imply endorsement of this article's contents, product, or anything else. Quote.

Bożek A, Nowak PF, Blukacz M. The Relationship Between Spirituality, Health-Related Behavior, and Psychological Well-Being. Front Psychol. 2020 Aug 14;11:1997. doi: 10.3389/fpsyg.2020.01997. PMID: 32922340; PMCID: PMC7457021. Copyright © 2020 Bożek, Nowak and Blukacz. This is an open-access article distributed under the terms of the Creative Commons Attribution License (CC BY). Reworded.

https://www.cdc.gov/pcd/issues/2016/15_0501.htm

https://www.nih.gov/news-events/news-releases/nih-awards-170-million-precision-nutrition-study

https://www.who.int/news-room/feature-stories/detail/traditional-medicine-has-a-long-history-of-contributing-to-conventional-medicine

https://www.nih.gov/health-information/nih-clinical-research-trials-you/finding-clinical-trial

http://nccam.nih.gov/health

Olliaro P, Torreele E. Managing the risks of making the wrong diagnosis: First, do no harm. Int J Infect Dis. 2021 May;106:382-385. doi: 10.1016/j.ijid.2021.04.004. Epub 2021 Apr 15. PMID: 33845195; PMCID: PMC8752462. © 2021 The Authors This is an open access article under the CC BY license (http://creativecommons.org/licenses/by/4.0/. Quote.

Alamri SS, Alsaieedi A, Khouqeer Y, Afeef M, Alharbi S, Algaissi A, Alghanmi M, Altorki T, Zawawi A, Alfaleh MA, Hashem AM, Alhabbab R. The importance of combining serological testing with RT-PCR assays for efficient detection of COVID-19 and higher diagnostic accuracy. *PeerJ*. 2023 Apr 11;11:e15024. doi: 10.7717/peerj.15024. PMID: 37065688; PMCID: PMC10103696. ©2023 Alamri et al. This is an open access article distributed under the terms of the **Creative Commons Attribution License.** Quote.

Ibid, reworded.

Patient Involvement in Health Care Decision Making: A Review Shaghayegh Vahdat, Leila Hamzehgardeshi, Somayeh Hessam, Zeinab Hamzehgardeshi *Iran Red Crescent Med J*. 2014 Jan; 16(1): e12454. Published online 2014 Jan 5. doi: 10.5812/ircmj.12454 PMCID: PMC3964421 Copyright © 2014, Iranian Red Crescent Medical Journal; Published by Kowsar Corp. This is an open-access article distributed under the terms of the Creative Commons Attribution License. Reworded

www.fda.gov/medwatch/report.htm

Yuan X, Wang N, Geng H, Zhang S. Mentalizing Another's Visual World-A Novel Exploration via Motion Aftereffect. *Front Psychol*. 2017 Sep 7;8:1535. doi: 10.3389/fpsyg.2017.01535. PMID: 28936191; PMCID: PMC5594217. Copyright © 2017 Yuan, Wang, Geng and Zhang. This is an open-access article distributed under the terms of the Creative Commons Attribution License (CC BY). Reworded.

www.fda.gov/medwatch/report.htm

First, Do No Harm (Gone Wrong): Total-Scale Analysis of Medical Errors Scientific Literature. *Front Public Health*. 2020 Oct 16;8:558913. doi: 10.3389/fpubh.2020.558913. PMID: 33178657; PMCID: PMC7596242. Copyright © 2020 Atanasov, Yeung, Klager, Eibensteiner, Schaden, Kletecka-Pulker and Willschke. Copyright © 2020 Atanasov, Yeung, Klager, Eibensteiner, Schaden, Kletecka-Pulker and Willschke. This is an open-access article distributed under the terms of the Creative Commons Attribution License (CC BY). Reworded.

Serafini B, Rosicarelli B, Veroni C, Mazzola GA, Aloisi F. Epstein-Barr Virus-Specific CD8 T Cells Selectively Infiltrate the Brain in Multiple Sclerosis and Interact Locally with Virus-Infected Cells: Clue for a Virus-Driven Immunopathological Mechanism. *J Virol*. 2019 Nov 26;93(24):e00980-19. doi: 10.1128/JVI.00980-19. PMID: 31578295; PMCID: PMC6880158. Copyright © 2019 Serafini et al. This is an open-access article distributed under the terms of the **Creative Commons Attribution 4.0 International license.** Reworded.

https://www.nih.gov/news-events/news-releases/nih-launches-clinical-trial-epstein-barr-virus-vaccine

**Chapter 6: Constituents of Disease Pathology**

https://www.cdc.gov/niosh/learning/safetyculturehc/module-2/3.html

Shimonovich M, Pearce A, Thomson H, Keyes K, Katikireddi SV. Assessing causality in epidemiology: revisiting Bradford Hill to incorporate developments in causal thinking. *Eur J Epidemiol. 2021* Sep;36(9):873-887. doi: 10.1007/s10654-020-00703-7. Epub 2020 Dec 16. PMID: 33324996; PMCID: PMC8206235. © The Author(s) 2020 Open Access. This article is licensed under a Creative Commons Attribution 4.0 International License. To view a copy of this licence, visit http://creativecommons.org/licenses/by/4.0/. Reworded.

Casamassimi A, Ciccodicola A, Rienzo M. Transcriptional Regulation and Its Misregulation in Human Diseases. *Int J Mol Sci.* 2023 May 12;24(10):8640. doi: 10.3390/ijms24108640. PMID: 37239985; PMCID: PMC10218156. © 2023 by the authors. Licensee MDPI, Basel, Switzerland. This article is an open access article distributed under the terms and conditions of the Creative Commons Attribution (CC BY) license (https://creativecommons.org/licenses/by/4.0/). Reworded.

Kirichenko TV, Markina YV, Bogatyreva AI, Tolstik TV, Varaeva YR, Starodubova AV. The Role of Adipokines in Inflammatory Mechanisms of Obesity. *Int J Mol Sci.* 2022 Nov 29;23(23):14982. doi: 10.3390/ijms232314982. PMID: 36499312; PMCID: PMC9740598. © 2022 by the authors. Licensee MDPI, Basel, Switzerland. This article is an open access article distributed under the terms and conditions of the Creative Commons Attribution (CC BY). License (https://creativecommons.org/licenses/by/4.0/). Reworded.

Lin X, Li H. Obesity: Epidemiology, Pathophysiology, and Therapeutics. *Front Endocrinol* (Lausanne). 2021 Sep 6;12:706978. doi: 10.3389/fendo.2021.706978. PMID: 34552557; PMCID: PMC8450866. Copyright © 2021 Lin and Li. This is an open-access article distributed under the terms of the Creative Commons Attribution License (CC BY). Reworded.

Knezevic E, Nenic K, Milanovic V, Knezevic NN. The Role of Cortisol in Chronic Stress, Neurodegenerative Diseases, and Psychological Disorders. *Cells.* 2023 Nov 29;12(23):2726. doi: 10.3390/cells12232726. PMID: 38067154; PMCID: PMC10706127. © 2023 by the authors. Licensee MDPI, Basel, Switzerland. This article is an open access article distributed

Wazir H, Abid M, Essani B, Saeed H, Ahmad Khan M, Nasrullah F, Qadeer U, Khalid A, Varrassi G, Muzammil MA, Maryam A, Syed ARS, Shah AA, Kinger S, Ullah F. Diagnosis and Treatment of Liver Disease: Current Trends and Future Directions. *Cureus*. 2023 Dec 4;15(12):e49920. doi: 10.7759/cureus.49920. PMID: 38174191; PMCID: PMC10763979. Copyright © 2023, Wazir et al. This is an open access article distributed under the terms of the Creative Commons Attribution License CC-BY 4.0. Reworded.

Sarmiento-Andrade Y, Suárez R, Quintero B, Garrochamba K, Chapela SP. Gut microbiota and obesity: New insights. *Front Nutr*. 2022 Oct 14;9:1018212. doi: 10.3389/fnut.2022.1018212. PMID: 36313072; PMCID: PMC9614660. Copyright © 2022 Sarmiento-Andrade, Suárez, Quintero, Garrochamba and Chapela. Creative Commons Attribution License (CC BY). Reworded.

Ibid, Lin & Li, 2021, reworded.

Taniya MA, Chung HJ, Al Mamun A, Alam S, Aziz MA, Emon NU, Islam MM, Hong SS, Podder BR, Ara Mimi A, Aktar Suchi S, Xiao J. Role of Gut Microbiome in Autism Spectrum Disorder and Its Therapeutic Regulation. *Front Cell Infect Microbiol*. 2022 Jul 22;12:915701. doi: 10.3389/fcimb.2022.915701. PMID: 35937689; PMCID: PMC9355470. Copyright © 2022 Taniya, Chung, Al Mamun, Alam, Aziz, Emon, Islam, Hong, Podder, Ara Mimi, Aktar Suchi and Xiao This is an open-access article distributed under the terms of the Creative Commons Attribution License (CC BY). Reworded.

Guskjolen A, Cembrowski MS. Engram neurons: Encoding, consolidation, retrieval, and forgetting of memory. Mol Psychiatry. 2023 Aug;28(8):3207-3219. doi: 10.1038/s41380-023-02137-5. Epub 2023 Jun 28. PMID: 37369721; PMCID: PMC10618102. © The Author(s) 2023. This article is licensed under a Creative Commons Attribution 4.0 International License, http://creativecommons.org/licenses/by/4.0/. Quote.

Dahiya D, Nigam PS. Antibiotic-Therapy-Induced Gut Dysbiosis Affecting Gut Microbiota-Brain Axis and Cognition: Restoration by Intake of Probiotics and Synbiotics. *Int J Mol Sci*. 2023 Feb 4;24(4):3074. doi: 10.3390/ijms24043074. PMID: 36834485; PMCID: PMC9959899. © 2023 by the authors. Licensee MDPI, Basel, Switzerland. This article is an open access article distributed under the terms and conditions of the Creative Commons Attribution (CC BY) license (https://creativecommons.org/licenses/by/4.0/. Reworded.

Zhang S, Lu S, Li Z. Extrahepatic factors in hepatic immune regulation. *Front Immunol.* 2022 Aug 16;13:941721. doi: 10.3389/fimmu.2022.941721. PMID: 36052075; PMCID: PMC9427192. Copyright © 2022 Zhang, Lu and Li. Creative Commons Attribution License (CC BY). Quote.

Sears B, Ricordi C. Anti-inflammatory nutrition as a pharmacological approach to treat obesity. J Obes. 2011;2011:431985. doi: 10.1155/2011/431985. Epub 2010 Sep 30. PMID: 20953366; PMCID: PMC2952901. Copyright © 2011 B. Sears and C. Ricordi. Copyright © 2011 B. Sears and C. Ricordi. This is an open access article distributed under the Creative Commons Attribution License. Quote.

Lelou E, Corlu A, Nesseler N, Rauch C, Mallédant Y, Seguin P, Aninat C. The Role of Catecholamines in Pathophysiological Liver Processes. *Cells.* 2022 Mar 17;11(6):1021. doi: 10.3390/cells11061021. PMID: 35326472; PMCID: PMC8947265. © 2022 by the authors. Licensee MDPI, Basel, Switzerland. This article is an open access article distributed under the terms and conditions of the Creative Commons Attribution (CC BY) license (https://creativecommons.org/licenses/by/4.0/. Reworded.

Yang Zhou J. Innate immunity and early liver inflammation. *Front Immunol.* 2023 May 2;14:1175147. doi: 10.3389/fimmu.2023.1175147. PMID: 37205101; PMCID: PMC10187146. Copyright © 2023 Yang Zhou. This is an open-access article distributed under the terms of the Creative Commons Attribution License (CC BY). Reworded.

Zhou M, Zhao X, Liao L, Deng Y, Liu M, Wang J, Xue X, Li Y. Forsythiaside A Regulates Activation of Hepatic Stellate Cells by Inhibiting NOX4-Dependent ROS. *Oxid Med Cell Longev.* 2022 Jan 5;2022:9938392. doi: 10.1155/2022/9938392. PMID: 35035671; PMCID: PMC8754607. Copyright © 2022 Mengting Zhou et al. This is an open access article distributed under the Creative Commons Attribution License. Reworded.

Blas-García A, Apostolova N. Novel Therapeutic Approaches to Liver Fibrosis Based on Targeting Oxidative Stress. *Antioxidants* (Basel). 2023 Aug 5;12(8):1567. doi: 10.3390/antiox12081567. PMID: 37627562; PMCID: PMC10451738. © 2023 by the authors. Licensee MDPI, Basel, Switzerland. This article is an open access article distributed under the terms and conditions of the Creative Commons Attribution (CC BY) license (https://creativecommons.org/licenses/by/4.0/. Reworded.

livertox.nih.gov (quote).

Llorente, C., Jepsen, P., Inamine, T. et al. Gastric acid suppression promotes alcoholic liver disease by inducing overgrowth of intestinal Enterococcus. *Nat Commun* 8, 837 (2017). https://doi.org/10.1038/s41467-017-00796-x. © The Author(s) 2017 Open Access. This article is licensed To view a copy of this license, visit http://creativecommons.org/licenses/by/4.0. Reworded.

Ibid, reworded.

Mega A, Marzi L, Kob M, Piccin A, Floreani A. Food and Nutrition in the Pathogenesis of Liver Damage. *Nutrients.* 2021 Apr 16;13(4):1326. doi: 10.3390/nu13041326. PMID: 33923822; PMCID: PMC8073814. © 2021 by the authors. Licensee MDPI, Basel, Switzerland. This article is an open access article distributed under the terms and conditions of the Creative Commons Attribution (CC BY) license (https://creativecommons.org/licenses/by/4.0/). Partial quote.

Singh DN, Bohra JS, Dubey TP, Shivahre PR, Singh RK, Singh T, Jaiswal DK. Common foods for boosting human immunity: A review. *Food Sci Nutr.* 2023 Aug 18;11(11):6761-6774. doi: 10.1002/fsn3.3628. PMID: 37970422; PMCID: PMC10630845. © 2023 The Authors. Food Science & Nutrition published by Wiley Periodicals LLC. This is an open access article under the terms of the http://creativecommons.org/licenses/by/4.0/. Reworded.

Singh et al., ibid, quote.

Singh, et al., ibid, reworded.

Costello E, Rock S, Stratakis N, Eckel SP, Walker DI, Valvi D, Cserbik D, Jenkins T, Xanthakos SA, Kohli R, Sisley S, Vasiliou V, La Merrill MA, Rosen H, Conti DV, McConnell R, Chatzi L. Exposure to per- and Polyfluoroalkyl Substances and Markers of Liver Injury: A Systematic Review and Meta-Analysis. *Environ Health Perspect.* 2022 Apr;130(4):46001. doi: 10.1289/EHP10092. Epub 2022 Apr 27. PMID: 35475652; PMCID: PMC9044977. *EHP* is an open-access journal published with support from the National Institute of Environmental Health Sciences, National Institutes of Health. All content is public domain unless otherwise noted. Reworded.

https://www.epa.gov/pfas/pfas-strategic-roadmap-epas-commitments-action-2021-2024#year-one-report

Singh S, Kola P, Kaur D, et al. Therapeutic Potential of Nutraceuticals and Dietary Supplements in the Prevention of Viral Diseases: A Review. *Front Nutr.* 2021;8:679312. Published 2021 Sep 17. doi:10.3389/fnut.2021.679312s. Copyright © 2021 Singh, Kola, Kaur, Singla, Mishra, Panesar, Mallikarjunan and Krishania. This is an open-access article distributed under the terms of the Creative Commons Attribution License (CC BY). Reworded. Reworded.

Ibid, Singh et al., 2021, reworded.

Ibid, Singh et al., 2021, reworded.

Chen J, Huang XF, Shao R, Chen C, Deng C. Molecular Mechanisms of Antipsychotic Drug-Induced Diabetes. *Front Neurosci*. 2017 Nov 21;11:643. doi: 10.3389/fnins.2017.00643. PMID: 29209160; PMCID: PMC5702456. Copyright © 2017 Chen, Huang, Shao, Chen and Deng. This is an open-access article distributed under the terms of the Creative Commons Attribution License (CC BY) Reworded CC 4.0. Partial quote.

Egalini F, Marinelli L, Rossi M, Motta G, Prencipe N, Rossetto Giaccherino R, Pagano L, Grottoli S, Giordano R. Endocrine disrupting chemicals: effects on pituitary, thyroid and adrenal glands. Endocrine. 2022 Dec;78(3):395-405. doi: 10.1007/s12020-022-03076-x. Epub 2022 May 23. PMID: 35604630; PMCID: PMC9637063. © The Author(s) 2022. This article is licensed under a Creative Commons Attribution 4.0 International License. Quote.

Guarnotta V, Tomasello L, Giordano C. Prediction of diabetes mellitus induced by steroid overtreatment in adrenal insufficiency. *Sci Rep*. 2022 Jan 18;12(1):885. doi: 10.1038/s41598-022-04904-w. PMID: 35042934; PMCID: PMC8766568. © 2022 by the authors. Licensee MDPI, Basel, Switzerland. This article is an open access article distributed under the terms and conditions of the Creative Commons Attribution (CC BY) license Reworded (https://creativecommons.org/licenses/by/4.0/). Quote.

Haidar Z, Fatema K, Shoily SS, Sajib AA. Disease-associated metabolic pathways affected by heavy metals and metalloid. *Toxicol Rep*. 2023 Apr 24;10:554-570. doi: 10.1016/j.toxrep.2023.04.010. PMID: 37396849; PMCID: PMC10313886. © 2023 The Authors. This is an open access article under the CC BY license (http://creativecommons.org/licenses/by/4.0/). Quote.

Ibid, reworded.

Lu S, Wei F, Li G. The evolution of the concept of stress and the framework of the stress system. *Cell Stress*. 2021 Apr 26;5(6):76-85. doi: 10.15698/cst2021.06.250. PMID: 34124582; PMCID: PMC8166217. Copyright: © 2021 Lu et al. Copyright: © 2021 Lu et al. This is an open-access article released under the terms of the Creative Commons Attribution (CC BY) license. Quote.

Ibid, reworded.

Quick JC, Henderson DF. Occupational Stress: Preventing Suffering, Enhancing Wellbeing. *Int J Environ Res Public Health*. 2016 Apr 29;13(5):459. doi: 10.3390/ijerph13050459. PMID: 27136575; PMCID: PMC4881084. © 2016 by the authors; licensee MDPI, Basel, Switzerland. © 2016 by the authors; licensee MDPI, Basel, Switzerland. This article is an open access article distributed under the terms and conditions of the Creative Commons Attribution (CC-BY) license (http://creativecommons.org/licenses/by/4.0. Reworded.

Ibid, quote.

Vandamme C, Kinnunen T. B cell helper T cells and type 1 diabetes. *Scand J Immunol.* 2020 Oct;92(4):e12943. doi: 10.1111/sji.12943. PMID: 32697399; PMCID: PMC7583378. © 2020 The Authors. *Scandinavian Journal of Immunology* published by John Wiley & Sons Ltd on behalf of The Scandinavian Foundation for Immunology. This is an open access article under the terms of the http://creativecommons.org/licenses/by/4.0/. Reworded.

Dinić S, Arambašić Jovanović J, Uskoković A, Mihailović M, Grdović N, Tolić A, Rajić J, Đorđević M, Vidaković M. Oxidative stress-mediated beta cell death and dysfunction as a target for diabetes management. *Front Endocrinol* (Lausanne). 2022 Sep 23;13:1006376. doi: 10.3389/fendo.2022.1006376. PMID: 36246880; PMCID: PMC9554708. Copyright © 2022 Dinić, Arambašić Jovanović, Uskoković, Mihailović, Grdović, Tolić, Rajić, Đorđević and Vidaković. Creative Commons Attribution License (CC BY) Quote.

Iatcu CO, Steen A, Covasa M. Gut Microbiota and Complications of Type-2 Diabetes. *Nutrients*. 2021 Dec 30;14(1):166. doi: 10.3390/nu14010166. PMID: 35011044; PMCID: PMC8747253. © 2021 by the authors. Licensee MDPI, Basel, Switzerland. This article is an open access article distributed under the terms and conditions of the Creative Commons Attribution (CC BY) license (https://creativecommons.org/licenses/by/4.0. Reworded.

Isaacs SR, Foskett DB, Maxwell AJ, Ward EJ, Faulkner CL, Luo JYX, Rawlinson WD, Craig ME, Kim KW. Viruses and Type 1 Diabetes: From Enteroviruses to the Virome. *Microorganisms*. 2021 Jul 16;9(7):1519. doi: 10.3390/microorganisms9071519. PMID: 34361954; PMCID: PMC8306446. © 2021 by the authors. Licensee MDPI, Basel, Switzerland. This article is an open access article distributed under the terms and conditions of the Creative Commons Attribution (CC BY) license (https://creativecommons.org/licenses/by/4.0/. Reworded.

Ibid, Isaacs et al, citing authors Couper et al., 2018 and Steck & Rewers, 2011, reworded.

Ibid, Issacs et al., 2021, quote.

Ibid, Issacs et al., 2021, quote

Nekoua MP, Mercier A, Alhazmi A, Sane F, Alidjinou EK, Hober D. Fighting Enteroviral Infections to Prevent Type 1 Diabetes. *Microorganisms.* 2022 Apr 1;10(4):768. doi: 10.3390/microorganisms10040768. PMID: 35456818; PMCID: PMC9031364. © 2022 by the authors. Licensee MDPI, Basel, Switzerland. This article is an open access article distributed under the terms and conditions of the Creative Commons Attribution (CC BY) license (https://creativecommons.org/licenses/by/4.0/). Quote.

Trinh QD. Recent Research in Cell Stress and Microbial Infection. *Microorganisms.* 2022 Mar 14;10(3):622. doi: 10.3390/microorganisms10030622. PMID: 35336195; PMCID: PMC8951272. © 2022 by the authors. Licensee MDPI, Basel, Switzerland. This article is an open access article distributed under the terms and conditions of the Creative Commons Attribution (CC BY) license (https://creativecommons.org/licenses/by/4.0. Reworded.

Fevang B, Wyller VBB, Mollnes TE, Pedersen M, Asprusten TT, Michelsen A, Ueland T, Otterdal K. Lasting Immunological Imprint of Primary Epstein-Barr Virus Infection With Associations to Chronic Low-Grade Inflammation and Fatigue. *Front Immunol.* 2021 Dec 20;12:715102. doi: 10.3389/fimmu.2021.715102. PMID: 34987499; PMCID: PMC8721200. Copyright © 2021 Fevang, Wyller, Mollnes, Pedersen, Asprusten, Michelsen, Ueland and Otterdal This is an open-access article distributed under the terms of the Creative Commons Attribution License (CC BY) Reworded.

Wang Y, Zhang M, Xue Q, Zhou H, Chen J, Wang H, Zhang Y, Shi W. Case report: Immune modulation after PD-1 inhibitor therapy in a patient with extranodal NK/T-cell lymphoma secondary to chronic active Epstein-Barr virus disease unveiled by single-cell transcriptomics. *Front Immunol.* 2023 Apr 17;14:1172307. doi: 10.3389/fimmu.2023.1172307. PMID: 37138889; PMCID: PMC10149821. Copyright © 2023 Wang, Zhang, Xue, Zhou, Chen, Wang, Zhang and Shi This is an open-access article distributed under the terms of the Creative Commons Attribution License (CC BY) Reworded.

Zhang YJ, Gan RY, Li S, Zhou Y, Li AN, Xu DP, Li HB. Antioxidant Phytochemicals for the Prevention and Treatment of Chronic Diseases. *Molecules.* 2015 Nov 27;20(12):21138-56. doi: 10.3390/molecules201219753. PMID: 26633317; PMCID: PMC6331972.

© 2015 by the authors. Licensee MDPI, Basel, Switzerland. This article is an open access article distributed under the terms and conditions of the Creative Commons by Attribution (CC-BY) license. Reworded.

Jiang S, Liu H, Li C. Dietary Regulation of Oxidative Stress in Chronic Metabolic Diseases. *Foods.* 2021 Aug 11;10(8):1854. doi: 10.3390/foods10081854. PMID: 34441631; PMCID: PMC8391153. © 2021 by the authors. Licensee MDPI, Basel, Switzerland. This article is an open access article distributed under the terms and conditions of the Creative Commons Attribution (CC BY) license (https://creativecommons.org/licenses/by/4.0/. Reworded.

Ibid, Jian et al., 2021, reworded.

Kleinman A, Benson P. Anthropology in the clinic: the problem of cultural competency and how to fix it. *PLoS Med.* 2006;3(10):e294. doi:10.1371/journal.pmed.0030294 © 2006 Kleinman and Benson. © 2006 Kleinman and Benson. This is an open-access article distributed under the terms of the Creative Commons Attribution License. Reworded.

Rao TS, Asha MR, Jagannatha Rao KS, Vasudevaraju P. The biochemistry of belief. *Indian J Psychiatry.* 2009 Oct-Dec;51(4):239-41. doi: 10.4103/0019-5545.58285. PMID: 20048445; PMCID: PMC2802367. © Indian Journal of Psychiatry. This is an open-access article distributed under the terms of the Creative Commons Attribution License. Quote.

*Epigenetics, Consciousness, & Reprogramming the Mind* - Dr Bruce Lipton, April 11, 2024, https://www.youtube.com/watch?v=FZexbpHLc_g

Ciążyńska M, Olejniczak-Staruch I, Sobolewska-Sztychny D, Narbutt J, Skibińska M, Lesiak A. Ultraviolet Radiation and Chronic Inflammation-Molecules and Mechanisms Involved in Skin Carcinogenesis: A Narrative Review. *Life (Basel).* 2021 Apr 8;11(4):326. doi: 10.3390/life11040326. PMID: 33917793; PMCID: PMC8068112. © 2021 by the authors. Licensee MDPI, Basel, Switzerland. This article is an open access article distributed under the terms and conditions of the Creative Commons Attribution (CC BY) license (https://creativecommons.org/licenses/by/4.0. Reworded.

Kany S, Vollrath JT, Relja B. Cytokines in Inflammatory Disease. *Int J Mol Sci.* 2019 Nov 28;20(23):6008. doi: 10.3390/ijms20236008. PMID: 31795299; PMCID: PMC6929211. © 2019 by the authors. Licensee MDPI, Basel, Switzerland. This article is an open access article distributed under the terms and conditions of the Creative Commons Attribution (CC BY) license (http://creativecommons.org/licenses/by/4.0. Quote.

Klein JR. Dynamic Interactions Between the Immune System and the Neuroendocrine System in Health and Disease. *Front Endocrinol* (Lausanne).

2021 Mar 22;12:655982. doi: 10.3389/fendo.2021.655982. PMID: 33828532; PMCID: PMC8020567. Copyright © 2021 Klein This is an open-access article distributed under the terms of the Creative Commons Attribution License (CC BY). Reworded.

Kunnumakkara AB, Sailo BL, Banik K, Harsha C, Prasad S, Gupta SC, Bharti AC, Aggarwal BB. Chronic diseases, inflammation, and spices: how are they linked? *J Transl Med.* 2018 Jan 25;16(1):14. doi: 10.1186/s12967-018-1381-2. PMID: 29370858; PMCID: PMC5785894. © The Author(s) 2018. This article is distributed under the terms of the Creative Commons Attribution 4.0 International License. http://creativecommons.org/publicdomain/zero/1.0/ The use of all articles cited within this text and end notes does not imply endorsement of any article contents, product, or anything else. Quote.

Ibid, Kunnumakkara et al., 2018, quote.

Ibid, Kunnumakkara et al., 2018, reworded.

Carr AC, Maggini S. Vitamin C and Immune Function. *Nutrients.* 2017 Nov 3;9(11):1211. doi: 10.3390/nu9111211. PMID: 29099763; PMCID: PMC5707683. © 2017 by the authors. Licensee MDPI, Basel, Switzerland. This article is an open access article distributed under the terms and conditions of the Creative Commons Attribution (CC BY) license (http://creativecommons.org/licenses/by/4.0/. Quote.

Islam R, Pupovac A, Evtimov V, Boyd N, Shu R, Boyd R, Trounson A. Enhancing a Natural Killer: Modification of NK Cells for Cancer Immunotherapy. *Cells.* 2021 Apr 29;10(5):1058. doi: 10.3390/cells10051058. PMID: 33946954; PMCID: PMC8146003. © 2021 by the authors. Licensee MDPI, Basel, Switzerland. This article is an open access article distributed under the terms and conditions of the Creative Commons Attribution (CC BY) license. CC 4.0. Reworded.

Welsh JA, Braun H, Brown N, Um C, Ehret K, Figueroa J, Boyd Barr D. Production-related contaminants (pesticides, antibiotics and hormones) in organic and conventionally produced milk samples sold in the USA. *Public Health Nutr.* 2019 Nov;22(16):2972-2980. doi: 10.1017/S136898001900106X. Epub 2019 Jun 26. PMID: 31238996; PMCID: PMC6792142 © The Authors 2019. This is an Open Access article, distributed under the terms of the Creative Commons Attribution license (http://creativecommons.org/licenses/by/4.0/. Quote.

Ciaunica A, Shmeleva EV, Levin M. The brain is not mental! coupling neuronal and immune cellular processing in human organisms. *Front Integr Neurosci.* 2023 May 17;17:1057622. doi: 10.3389/fnint.2023.1057622. PMID: 37265513; PMCID: PMC10230067. Copyright © 2023 Ciaunica,

Shmeleva and Levin. This is an open-access article distributed under the terms of the Creative Commons Attribution License (CC BY). Quote.

Ibid, Ciaunica et al., 2023, quote.

Baluška F, Miller WB Jr, Reber AS. Biomolecular Basis of Cellular Consciousness via Subcellular Nanobrains. *Int J Mol Sci.* 2021 Mar 3;22(5):2545. doi: 10.3390/ijms22052545. PMID: 33802617; PMCID: PMC7961929. © 2021 by the authors. Licensee MDPI, Basel, Switzerland. This article is an open access article distributed under the terms and conditions of the Creative Commons Attribution (CC BY) license (http://creativecommons.org/licenses/by/4.0. Quote.

Ibid, Baluška et al., 2021, quote.

Odularu AT, Afolayan AJ, Sadimenko AP, Ajibade PA, Mbese JZ. Multidrug-Resistant Biofilm, Quorum Sensing, Quorum Quenching, and Antibacterial Activities of Indole Derivatives as Potential Eradication Approaches. *Biomed Res Int.* 2022 Aug 24;2022:9048245. doi: 10.1155/2022/9048245. PMID: 36060142; PMCID: PMC9433265. Copyright © 2022 Ayodele T. Odularu et al. This is an open access article distributed under the Creative Commons Attribution License, which permits unrestricted use, distribution, and reproduction in any medium, provided the original work is properly cited. Quote.

Esteve M. Mechanisms Underlying Biological Effects of Cruciferous Glucosinolate-Derived Isothiocyanates/Indoles: A Focus on Metabolic Syndrome. *Front Nutr.* 2020 Sep 2;7:111. doi: 10.3389/fnut.2020.00111. PMID: 32984393; PMCID: PMC7492599. Copyright © 2020 Esteve. This is an open-access article distributed under the terms of the Creative Commons Attribution License (CC BY). Reworded.

Chakrabarti A, Geurts L, Hoyles L, Iozzo P, Kraneveld AD, La Fata G, Miani M, Patterson E, Pot B, Shortt C, Vauzour D. The microbiota-gut-brain axis: pathways to better brain health. Perspectives on what we know, what we need to investigate and how to put knowledge into practice. *Cell Mol Life Sci.* 2022 Jan 19;79(2):80. doi: 10.1007/s00018-021-04060-w. PMID: 35044528; PMCID: PMC8770392. © The Author(s) 2022 Open Access. This article is licensed under a Creative Commons Attribution 4.0 International Licens., To view a copy of this license, visit http://creativecommons.org/licenses/by/4.0. Reworded.

Patangia DV, Anthony Ryan C, Dempsey E, Paul Ross R, Stanton C. Impact of antibiotics on the human microbiome and consequences for host health. *Microbiologyopen.* 2022 Feb;11(1):e1260. doi: 10.1002/mbo3.1260. PMID: 35212478; PMCID: PMC8756738. © 2021 The Authors. *MicrobiologyOpen* published by John Wiley & Sons Ltd. © 2021.

This is an open access article under the terms of the http://creativecommons.org/licenses/by/4.0/. Reworded.

Ibid, Chakrabarti, et al., 2022, reworded.

Ye J, Wu Z, Zhao Y, Zhang S, Liu W, Su Y. Role of gut microbiota in the pathogenesis and treatment of diabetes mullites: Advanced research-based review. *Front Microbiol*. 2022 Oct 19;13:1029890. doi: 10.3389/fmicb.2022.1029890. PMID: 36338058; PMCID: PMC9627042. Copyright © 2022 Ye, Wu, Zhao, Zhang, Liu and Su. This is an open-access article distributed under the terms of the Creative Commons Attribution License (CC BY). Reworded.

Kopacz K, Phadtare S. Probiotics for the Prevention of Antibiotic Associated Diarrhea. *Healthcare* (Basel). 2022 Aug 2;10(8):1450. doi: 10.3390/healthcare10081450. PMID: 36011108; PMCID: PMC9408191. © 2022 by the authors. Licensee MDPI, Basel, Switzerland. This article is an open access article distributed under the terms and conditions of the Creative Commons Attribution (CC BY) license (https://creativecommons.org/licenses/by/4.0/. Reworded.

Curty G, Marston JL, de Mulder Rougvie M, Leal FE, Nixon DF, Soares MA. Human Endogenous Retrovirus K in Cancer: A Potential Biomarker and Immunotherapeutic Target. *Viruses*. 2020;12(7):726. Published 2020 Jul 6. doi:10.3390/v12070726. © 2020 by the authors. Licensee MDPI, Basel, Switzerland. This article is an open access article distributed under the terms and conditions of the Creative Commons Attribution (CC BY) license (http://creativecommons.org/licenses/by/4.0. Quote.

Colon-Echevarria CB, Lamboy-Caraballo R, Aquino-Acevedo AN, Armaiz-Pena GN. Neuroendocrine Regulation of Tumor-Associated Immune Cells. *Front Oncol*. 2019 Oct 29;9:1077. doi: 10.3389/fonc.2019.01077. PMID: 31737559; PMCID: PMC682884 . Copyright © 2019 Colon-Echevarria, Lamboy-Caraballo, Aquino-Acevedo and Armaiz-Pena. This is an open-access article distributed under the terms of the Creative Commons Attribution License (CC BY). Quote.

Dai S, Mo Y, Wang Y, Xiang B, Liao Q, Zhou M, Li X, Li Y, Xiong W, Li G, Guo C, Zeng Z. Chronic Stress Promotes Cancer Development. *Front Oncol*. 2020 Aug 19;10:1492. doi: 10.3389/fonc.2020.01492. PMID: 32974180; PMCID: PMC7466429. Copyright © 2020 Dai, Mo, Wang, Xiang, Liao, Zhou, Li, Li, Xiong, Li, Guo and Zeng. This is an open-access article distributed under the terms of the Creative Commons Attribution License (CC BY). Reworded.

Rappaport SM. Genetic Factors Are Not the Major Causes of Chronic Diseases. *PLoS One*. 2016;11(4):e0154387. Published 2016 Apr 22. doi:10.1371/journal.pone.0154387. © 2016 Stephen M. Rappaport. This is an open access article distributed under the terms of the Creative Commons Attribution License. Quote.

Carter CS, Kingsbury MA. Oxytocin and oxygen: the evolution of a solution to the 'stress of life'. Philos Trans R Soc Lond B Biol Sci. 2022 Aug 29;377(1858):20210054. doi: 10.1098/rstb.2021.0054. Epub 2022 Jul 11. PMID: 35856299; PMCID: PMC9272143. © 2022 The Authors. Published by the Royal Society under the terms of the Creative Commons Attribution License http://creativecommons.org/licenses/by/4.0/. Reworded.

Sim M, Kim CS, Shon WJ, Lee YK, Choi EY, Shin DM. Hydrogen-rich water reduces inflammatory responses and prevents apoptosis of peripheral blood cells in healthy adults: a randomized, double-blind, controlled trial. *Sci Rep*. 2020 Jul 22;10(1):12130. doi: 10.1038/s41598-020-68930-2. PMID: 32699287; PMCID: PMC7376192. © The Author(s) 2020. CC 4.0. Reworded.

Münz C. Redirecting T Cells against Epstein-Barr Virus Infection and Associated Oncogenesis. *Cells*. 2020 Jun 4;9(6):1400. doi: 10.3390/cells9061400. PMID: 32512847; PMCID: PMC7349826. © 2020 by the author. Licensee MDPI, Basel, Switzerland. This article is an open access article distributed under the terms and conditions of the Creative Commons Attribution (CC BY) license (http://creativecommons.org/licenses/by/4.0/. Quote.

Ibid, Münz , 2020, quote.

Sawada A, Inoue M. Hematopoietic Stem Cell Transplantation for the Treatment of Epstein-Barr Virus-Associated T- or NK-Cell Lymphoproliferative Diseases and Associated Disorders. *Front Pediatr*. 2018 Nov 6;6:334. doi: 10.3389/fped.2018.00334. PMID: 30460216; PMCID: PMC6232123. Copyright © 2018 Sawada and Inoue. This is an open-access article distributed under the terms of the Creative Commons Attribution License (CC BY). Reworded.

Maydych V. The Interplay Between Stress, Inflammation, and Emotional Attention: Relevance for Depression. *Front Neurosci*. 2019 Apr 24;13:384. doi: 10.3389/fnins.2019.00384. PMID: 31068783; PMCID: PMC6491771. Copyright © 2019 Maydych. This is an open-access article distributed under the terms of the Creative Commons Attribution License (CC BY). Reworded.

Ibid, Maydych, 29019, reworded.

Wright CD, Tiani AG, Billingsley AL, Steinman SA, Larkin KT, McNeil DW. A Framework for Understanding the Role of Psychological Processes in Disease Development, Maintenance, and Treatment: The 3P-Disease Model. *Front Psychol*. 2019 Nov 20;10:2498. doi: 10.3389/fpsyg.2019.02498.

PMID: 31824367; PMCID: PMC6879427. Copyright © 2019 Wright, Tiani, Billingsley, Steinman, Larkin and McNeil. This is an open-access article distributed under the terms of the Creative Commons Attribution License (CC BY). Quote

Ibid, Maydych, 2019, quote

Ibid, Maydych, 2019, quote.

Liu YZ, Wang YX, Jiang CL. Inflammation: The Common Pathway of Stress-Related Diseases. *Front Hum Neurosci*. 2017 Jun 20;11:316. doi: 10.3389/fnhum.2017.00316. PMID: 28676747; PMCID: PMC5476783. Copyright © 2017 Liu, Wang and Jiang. This is an open-access article distributed under the terms of the Creative Commons Attribution License (CC BY). Reworded.

Ibid, Liu et al., 2017, reworded.

https://www.nimh.nih.gov/health/publications/looking-at-my-genes

Wiśniowiecka-Kowalnik B, Nowakowska BA. Genetics and epigenetics of autism spectrum disorder-current evidence in the field. J Appl Genet. 2019 Feb;60(1):37-47. doi: 10.1007/s13353-018-00480-w. Epub 2019 Jan 10. PMID: 30627967; PMCID: PMC6373410. © The Author(s) 2019. Open Access This article is distributed under the terms of the Creative Commons Attribution 4.0 International License. Reworded. (http://creativecommons.org/licenses/by/4.0/). Reworded.

Ding M, Shi S, Qie S, Li J, Xi X. Association between heavy metals exposure (cadmium, lead, arsenic, mercury) and child autistic disorder: a systematic review and meta-analysis. *Front Pediatr*. 2023 Jul 4;11:1169733. doi: 10.3389/fped.2023.1169733. PMID: 37469682; PMCID: PMC10353844. © 2023 Ding, Shi, Qie, Li and Xi. This is an open-access article distributed under the terms of the Creative Commons Attribution License (CC BY). Reworded.

Sampath VP, Singh SV, Pelov I, Tirosh O, Erel Y, Lichtstein D. Chemical Element Profiling in the Sera and Brain of Bipolar Disorders Patients and Healthy Controls. *Int J Mol Sci*. 2022 Nov 18;23(22):14362. doi: 10.3390/ijms232214362. PMID: 36430840; PMCID: PMC9692593. © 2022 by the authors. Licensee MDPI, Basel, Switzerland. This article is an open access article distributed under the terms and conditions of the Creative Commons Attribution (CC BY) license (https://creativecommons.org/licenses/by/4.0/ Reworded.

Lee YS, Ryu Y, Jung WM, Kim J, Lee T, Chae Y. Understanding Mind-Body Interaction from the Perspective of East Asian Medicine. *Evid Based*

*Complement Alternat Med.* 2017;2017:7618419. doi: 10.1155/2017/7618419. Epub 2017 Aug 22. PMID: 28904561; PMCID: PMC5585554. Copyright © 2017 Ye-Seul Lee et al. This is an open access article distributed under the Creative Commons Attribution License. Reworded.

https://www.cdc.gov/vitalsigns/aces/

https://www.cdc.gov/violenceprevention/aces

Herzog JI, Schmahl C. Adverse Childhood Experiences and the Consequences on Neurobiological, Psychosocial, and Somatic Conditions Across the Lifespan. *Front Psychiatry.* 2018;9:420. Published 2018 Sep 4. doi:10.3389/fpsyt.2018.00420. Copyright © 2018 Herzog and Schmahl. This is an open-access article distributed under the terms of the Creative Commons Attribution License (CC BY). Reworded.

www.cdc.gov/violenceprevention/pdf/brfss_adverse_module.pdf quote.

Pai A, Suris AM, North CS. Posttraumatic Stress Disorder in the DSM-5: Controversy, Change, and Conceptual Considerations. Behav Sci (Basel). 2017 Feb 13;7(1):7. doi: 10.3390/bs7010007. PMID: 28208816; PMCID: PMC5371751. © 2017 by the authors. Licensee MDPI, Basel, Switzerland. This article is an open access article distributed under the terms and conditions of the Creative Commons Attribution (CC BY) license (http://creativecommons.org/licenses/by/4.0/. Reworded.

Coventry PA, Meader N, Melton H, Temple M, Dale H, Wright K, Cloitre M, Karatzias T, Bisson J, Roberts NP, Brown JVE, Barbui C, Churchill R, Lovell K, McMillan D, Gilbody S. Psychological and pharmacological interventions for posttraumatic stress disorder and comorbid mental health problems following complex traumatic events: Systematic review and component network meta-analysis. *PLoS Med.* 2020 Aug 19;17(8):e1003262. doi: 10.1371/journal.pmed.1003262. PMID: 32813696; PMCID: PMC7446790. © 2020 Coventry et al. This is an open access article distributed under the terms of the Creative Commons Attribution License. Quote.

Zhu L, Li L, Li XZ, Wang L. Mind-Body Exercises for PTSD Symptoms, Depression, and Anxiety in Patients With PTSD: A Systematic Review and Meta-Analysis. *Front Psychol.* 2022 Jan 18;12:738211. doi: 10.3389/fpsyg.2021.738211. PMID: 35153889; PMCID: PMC8833099. Copyright © 2022 Zhu, Li, Li and Wang. This is an open-access article distributed under the terms of the Creative Commons Attribution License (CC BY). Reworded.

Ibid, Lee et al., 2017, reworded.

https://www.ptsd.va.gov.

private enterprise such as allsecurefoundation.org

Xia F, Li Q, Luo X, Wu J. Machine learning model for depression based on heavy metals among aging people: A study with National Health and Nutrition Examination Survey 2017-2018. *Front Public Health*. 2022 Aug 4;10:939758. doi: 10.3389/fpubh.2022.939758. PMID: 35991018; PMCID: PMC9386350. Copyright © 2022 Xia, Li, Luo and Wu. This is an open-access article distributed under the terms of the Creative Commons Attribution License (CC BY). Reworded.

Mikulska J, Juszczyk G, Gawrońska-Grzywacz M, Herbet M. HPA Axis in the Pathomechanism of Depression and Schizophrenia: New Therapeutic Strategies Based on Its Participation. *Brain Sci*. 2021 Sep 30;11(10):1298. doi: 10.3390/brainsci11101298. PMID: 34679364; PMCID: PMC8533829. © 2021 by the authors. Licensee MDPI, Basel, Switzerland. This article is an open access article distributed under the terms and conditions of the Creative Commons Attribution (CC BY) license. Reworded.

Ibid, Liu et al., 2017, reworded.

Pender MP. Hypothesis: bipolar disorder is an Epstein-Barr virus-driven chronic autoimmune disease - implications for immunotherapy. *Clin Transl Immunology*. 2020 Apr 6;9(4):e1116. doi: 10.1002/cti2.1116. PMID: 32257210; PMCID: PMC7133420. © 2020 The Authors. *Clinical & Translational Immunology* published by John Wiley & Sons Australia, Ltd on behalf of Australian and New Zealand Society for Immunology Inc. This is an open access article under the terms of the http://creativecommons.org/licenses/by/4.0/. Quote.

Pongratz G, Straub RH. The sympathetic nervous response in inflammation. *Arthritis Res Ther*. 2014;16(6):504. doi: 10.1186/s13075-014-0504-2. PMID: 25789375; PMCID: PMC4396833. © Pongratz and Straub; licensee BioMed Central Ltd. 2014. (http://creativecommons.org/publicdomain/zero/1.0/). The use of this article does not imply endorsement of this article's contents, product, or anything else. Quote.

Ibid, Pongratz & Straub 2014, quote.

Lee CH, Giuliani F. The Role of Inflammation in Depression and Fatigue. *Front Immunol*. 2019 Jul 19;10:1696. doi: 10.3389/fimmu.2019.01696. PMID: 31379879; PMCID: PMC6658985. Copyright © 2019 Lee and Giuliani. This is an open-access article distributed under the terms of the Creative Commons Attribution License (CC BY). Quote.

Quaglia M, Merlotti G, De Andrea M, Borgogna C, Cantaluppi V. Viral Infections and Systemic Lupus Erythematosus: New Players in an Old Story. *Viruses*. 2021 Feb 11;13(2):277. doi: 10.3390/v13020277. PMID:

33670195; PMCID: PMC7916951. © 2021 by the authors. Licensee MDPI, Basel, Switzerland. This article is an open access article distributed under the terms and conditions of the Creative Commons Attribution (CC BY) license (http://creativecommons.org/licenses/by/4.0/. Quote.

Moreno-Martinez L, Macías-Redondo S, Strunk M, Guillén-Antonini MI, Lunetta C, Tarlarini C, Penco S, Calvo AC, Osta R, Schoorlemmer J. New Insights into Endogenous Retrovirus-K Transcripts in Amyotrophic Lateral Sclerosis. *Int J Mol Sci.* 2024 Jan 26;25(3):1549. doi: 10.3390/ijms25031549. PMID: 38338823; PMCID: PMC10855536. © 2024 by the authors. Licensee MDPI, Basel, Switzerland. This article is an open access article distributed under the terms and conditions of the Creative Commons Attribution (CC BY) license (https://creativecommons.org/licenses/by/4.0/). Reworded.

Saha A, Robertson ES. Mechanisms of B-Cell Oncogenesis Induced by Epstein-Barr Virus. *J Virol.* 2019 Jun 14;93(13):e00238-19. doi: 10.1128/JVI.00238-19. PMID: 30971472; PMCID: PMC6580952. Copyright © 2019 Saha and Robertson. This is an open-access article distributed under the terms of the Creative Commons Attribution 4.0 International license. Reworded.

Fugl A, Andersen CL. Epstein-Barr virus and its association with disease – a review of relevance *Front Mol Biosci* to general practice. *BMC Fam Pract.* 2019 May 14;20(1):62. doi: 10.1186/s12875-019-0954-3. PMID: 31088382; PMCID: PMC6518816. © The Author(s). 2019. Open Access This article is distributed under the terms of the Creative Commons Attribution 4.0 International License (http://creativecommons.org/licenses/by/4.0/), (http://creativecommons.org/publicdomain/zero/1.0/). The use of this article cited within this article does not imply endorsement of any article contents, product, or anything else. Reworded.

Trier N, Izarzugaza J, Chailyan A, Marcatili P, Houen G. Human MHC-II with Shared Epitope Motifs Are Optimal Epstein-Barr Virus Glycoprotein 42 Ligands-Relation to Rheumatoid Arthritis. *Int J Mol Sci.* 2018;19(1):317. Published 2018 Jan 21. doi:10.3390/ijms19010317. © 2018 by the authors.Licensee MDPI, Basel, Switzerland. This article is an open access article distributed under the terms and conditions of the Creative Commons Attribution (CC BY) license (http://creativecommons.org/licenses/by/4.0. Reworded.

Jung YJ, Tweedie D, Scerba MT, Greig NH. Neuroinflammation as a Factor of Neurodegenerative Disease: Thalidomide Analogs as Treatments. *Front Cell Dev Biol.* 2019 Dec 4;7:313. doi: 10.3389/fcell.2019.00313. PMID: 31867326; PMCID: PMC6904283. Copyright © 2019 Jung, Tweedie, Scerba and Greig. This is an open-access article distributed under the terms of the Creative Commons Attribution License (CC BY). Reworded.

He R, Du Y, Wang C. Epstein-Barr virus infection: the leading cause of multiple sclerosis. Signal Transduct Target Ther. 2022 Jul 16;7(1):239. doi: 10.1038/s41392-022-01100-0. PMID: 35842414; PMCID: PMC9288537. © The Author(s) 2022. This article is licensed under a Creative Commons Attribution 4.0 International License, http://creativecommons.org/licenses/by/4.0/. Quote.

Hachim MY, Elemam NM, Maghazachi AA. The Beneficial and Debilitating Effects of Environmental and Microbial Toxins, Drugs, Organic Solvents and Heavy Metals on the Onset and Progression of Multiple Sclerosis. *Toxins* (Basel). 2019 Mar 5;11(3):147. doi: 10.3390/toxins11030147. PMID: 30841532; PMCID: PMC6468554. © 2019 by the authors. Licensee MDPI, Basel, Switzerland. This article is an open access article distributed under the terms and conditions of the Creative Commons Attribution (CC BY) license. Reworded.

Zhang N, Zuo Y, Jiang L, Peng Y, Huang X, Zuo L. Epstein-Barr Virus and Neurological Diseases. *Front Mol Biosci*. 2022 Jan 10;8:816098. doi: 10.3389/fmolb.2021.816098. PMID: 35083281; PMCID: PMC8784775. Copyright © 2022 Zhang, Zuo, Jiang, Peng, Huang and Zuo. Reworded. This is an open-access article distributed under the terms of the Creative Commons Attribution License (CC BY). Quote.

Sausen DG, Bhutta MS, Gallo ES, Dahari H, Borenstein R. Stress-Induced Epstein-Barr Virus Reactivation. *Biomolecules*. 2021 Sep 18;11(9):1380. doi: 10.3390/biom11091380. PMID: 34572593; PMCID: PMC8470332. © 2021 by the authors. Licensee MDPI, Basel, Switzerland. This article is an open access article distributed under the terms and conditions of the Creative Commons Attribution (CC BY) license (https://creativecommons.org/licenses/by/4.0/. Reworded.

Weider T, Genoni A, Broccolo F, Paulsen TH, Dahl-Jørgensen K, Toniolo A, Hammerstad SS. High Prevalence of Common Human Viruses in Thyroid Tissue. *Front Endocrinol* (Lausanne). 2022 Jul 14;13:938633. doi: 10.3389/fendo.2022.938633. PMID: 35909527; PMCID: PMC9333159. Copyright © 2022 Weider, Genoni, Broccolo, Paulsen, Dahl-Jørgensen, Toniolo and Hammerstad. This is an open-access article distributed under the terms of the Creative Commons Attribution License (CC BY). Reworded.

Yang T, Yang Y, Wang D, Li C, Qu Y, Guo J, Shi T, Bo W, Sun Z, Asakawa T. The clinical value of cytokines in chronic fatigue syndrome. *J Transl Med*. 2019 Jun 28;17(1):213. doi: 10.1186/s12967-019-1948-6. PMID: 31253154; PMCID: PMC6599310. © The Author(s) 2019. CC 4.0.* (http://creativecommons.org/publicdomain/zero/1.0/. Reworded. The use of all articles cited within this text and end notes does not imply endorsement of any article contents, product, or anything else. Reworded.

Lee JS, Kim HG, Lee DS, Son CG. Oxidative Stress is a Convincing Contributor to Idiopathic Chronic Fatigue. *Sci Rep*. 2018 Aug 27;8(1):12890. doi: 10.1038/s41598-018-31270-3. PMID: 30150620; PMCID: PMC6110864. © The Author(s) 2018. This article is licensed under a Creative Commons Attribution 4.0 International License. http://creativecommons.org/licenses/by/4.0/. Quote.

Tassinari R, Cavallini C, Olivi E, Facchin F, Taglioli V, Zannini C, Marcuzzi M, Ventura C. Cell Responsiveness to Physical Energies: Paving the Way to Decipher a Morphogenetic Code. *Int J Mol Sci*. 2022 Mar 15;23(6):3157. doi: 10.3390/ijms23063157. PMID: 35328576; PMCID: PMC8949133. © 2022 by the authors. Licensee MDPI, Basel, Switzerland. This article is an open access article distributed under the terms and conditions of the Creative Commons Attribution (CC BY) license. CC 4.0. Quote.

**Ibid, Tassinari et al., 2022, quote.**

Klimasiński M, Baum E, Praczyk J, Ziemkiewicz M, Springer D, Cofta S, Wieczorowska-Tobis K. Spiritual Distress and Spiritual Needs of Chronically Ill Patients in Poland: A Cross-Sectional Study. *Int J Environ Res Public Health*. 2022 May 1;19(9):5512. doi: 10.3390/ijerph19095512. PMID: 35564907; PMCID: PMC9101665. © 2022 by the authors. Licensee MDPI, Basel, Switzerland. This article is an open access article distributed under the terms and conditions of the Creative Commons Attribution (CC BY) license (https://creativecommons.org/licenses/by/4.0. Reworded.

Mendes BV, Donato SCT, Silva TLD, Penha RM, Jaman-Mewes P, Salvetti MG. Spiritual well-being, symptoms and performance of patients under palliative care. *Rev Bras Enferm*. 2023 Apr 7;76(2):e20220007. doi: 10.1590/0034-7167-2022-0007. PMID: 37042924; PMCID: PMC10084779. This is an Open Access article distributed under the terms of the Creative Commons Attribution License. Reworded.

Supplements to A Course in Miracles (ACIM, Suppl.Preface) ACIM IV. The Process of Illness, ACIM, P-2.IV.1:1-7 https://acim.org/acim/psychotherapy/the-process-of-illness/en/s/908

Jaishankar M, Tseten T, Anbalagan N, Mathew BB, Beeregowda KN. Toxicity, mechanism and health effects of some heavy metals. *Interdiscip Toxicol*. 2014;7(2):60-72. doi:10.2478/intox-2014-0009. Copyright © 2014 SETOX & Institute of Experimental Pharmacology and Toxicology, SASc. This is an open-access article distributed under the terms of the Creative Commons Attribution License. Quote.

Jan AT, Azam M, Siddiqui K, Ali A, Choi I, Haq QM. Heavy Metals and Human Health: Mechanistic Insight into Toxicity and Counter Defense System of Antioxidants. *Int J Mol Sci*. 2015;16(12):29592-29630. Published 2015 Dec 10. doi:10.3390/ijms161226183 PMID: 26690422; PMCID:

PMC4691126. © 2015 by the authors; licensee MDPI, Basel, Switzerland. This article is an open access article distributed under the terms and conditions of the Creative Commons by Attribution (CC-BY) license (http://creativecommons.org/licenses/by/4.0. Quote.

Zhang M, Liu T, Wang G, Buckley JP, Guallar E, Hong X, Wang MC, Wills-Karp M, Wang X, Mueller NT. *In Utero* Exposure to Heavy Metals and Trace Elements and Childhood Blood Pressure in a U.S. Urban, Low-Income, Minority Birth Cohort. *Environ Health Perspect*. 2021 Jun;129(6):67005. doi: 10.1289/EHP8325. Epub 2021 Jun 23. PMID: 34160246; PMCID: PMC8221032. *EHP* is an open-access journal published with support from the National Institute of Environmental Health Sciences, National Institutes of Health. All content is public domain unless otherwise noted. Reworded.

Balali-Mood M, Naseri K, Tahergorabi Z, Khazdair MR, Sadeghi M. Toxic Mechanisms of Five Heavy Metals: Mercury, Lead, Chromium, Cadmium, and Arsenic. Front Pharmacol. 2021 Apr 13;12:643972. doi: 10.3389/fphar.2021.643972. PMID: 33927623; PMCID: PMC8078867. Copyright © 2021 Balali-Mood, Naseri, Tahergorabi, Khazdair and Sadeghi.This is an open-access article distributed under the terms of the Creative Commons Attribution License (CC BY). Reworded.

Toni M, Massimino ML, De Mario A, Angiulli E, Spisni E. Metal Dyshomeostasis and Their Pathological Role in Prion and Prion-Like Diseases: The Basis for a Nutritional Approach. *Front Neurosci*. 2017 Jan 19;11:3. doi: 10.3389/fnins.2017.00003. PMID: 28154522; PMCID: PMC5243831. Copyright © 2017 Toni, Massimino, De Mario, Angiulli and Spisni. This is an open-access article distributed under the terms of the Creative Commons Attribution License (CC BY). Reworded.

Thakur M, Rachamalla M, Niyogi S, Datusalia AK, Flora SJS. Molecular Mechanism of Arsenic-Induced Neurotoxicity including Neuronal Dysfunctions. Int J Mol Sci. 2021 Sep 17;22(18):10077. doi: 10.3390/ijms221810077. PMID: 34576240; PMCID: PMC8471829. © 2021 by the authors. Licensee MDPI, Basel, Switzerland. This article is an open access article distributed under the terms and conditions of the Creative Commons Attribution (CC BY) license (https://creativecommons.org/licenses/by/4.0. Reworded.

Lee MJ, Chou MC, Chou WJ, Huang CW, Kuo HC, Lee SY, Wang LJ. Heavy Metals' Effect on Susceptibility to Attention-Deficit/Hyperactivity Disorder: Implication of Lead, Cadmium, and Antimony. *Int J Environ Res Public Health*. 2018 Jun 10;15(6):1221. doi: 10.3390/ijerph15061221. PMID: 29890770; PMCID: PMC6025252. © 2018 by the authors. Licensee MDPI, Basel, Switzerland. This article is an open access article distributed under the terms and conditions of the Creative Commons Attribution (CC BY) license (http://creativecommons.org/licenses/by/4.0/. Reworded.

Minich DM, Brown BI. A Review of Dietary (Phyto)Nutrients for Glutathione Support. *Nutrients*. 2019 Sep 3;11(9):2073. doi: 10.3390/nu11092073. PMID: 31484368; PMCID: PMC6770193. © 2019 by the authors. Licensee MDPI, Basel, Switzerland. This article is an open access article distributed under the terms and conditions of the Creative Commons Attribution (CC BY) license (http://creativecommons.org/licenses/by/4.0. Reworded.

Kontoghiorghes GJ. Advances on Chelation and Chelator Metal Complexes in Medicine. *Int J Mol Sci*. 2020 Apr 3;21(7):2499. doi: 10.3390/ijms21072499. PMID: 32260293; PMCID: PMC7177276. © 2020 by the author. Licensee MDPI, Basel, Switzerland. This article is an open access article distributed under the terms and conditions of the Creative Commons Attribution (CC BY) license (http://creativecommons.org/licenses/by/4.0/.

truthaboutfluoride.com/fluoride-detox.

Kopfler, F., H. Ringhand, W. Coleman, AND J. Meier. REACTIONS OF CHLORINE IN DRINKING WATER, WITH HUMIC ACIDS AND 'IN VIVO'. U.S. Environmental Protection Agency, Washington, D.C., EPA/600/D-84/196 (NTIS PB85160737).

Baby R, Hussein MZ, Abdullah AH, Zainal Z. Nanomaterials for the Treatment of Heavy Metal Contaminated Water. *Polymers* (Basel). 2022 Jan 31;14(3):583. doi: 10.3390/polym14030583. PMID: 35160572; PMCID: PMC8838446. © 2022 by the authors. Licensee MDPI, Basel, Switzerland. This article is an open access article distributed under the terms and conditions of the Creative Commons Attribution (CC BY) license (https://creativecommons.org/licenses/by/4.0/. Reworded.

https://www.fda.gov/food/food-additives-petitions/bisphenol-bpa-use-food-contact-application

Barrett JR. POPs vs. fat: persistent organic pollutant toxicity targets and is modulated by adipose tissue. *Environ Health Perspect*. 2013 Feb;121(2):a61. doi: 10.1289/ehp.121-a61. PMID: 23380189; PMCID: PMC3569705. Publication of EHP lies in the public domain and is therefore without copyright. All text from EHP may be reprinted freely. Use of materials published in EHP should be acknowledged. Reproduced with permission from Environmental Health Perspectives. Reworded.

https://beyondpesticides.org/dailynewsblog

Ibid, beyond pesticides.org

https://www.usgs.gov/news/new-study-identifies-pesticide-mixtures-us-rivers-and-streams

https://www.usgs.gov/centers/ohio-kentucky-indiana-water-science-center/science/pesticides.

Gunn CM, Sprague Martinez LS, Battaglia TA, Lobb R, Chassler D, Hakim D, Drainoni ML. Integrating community engagement with implementation science to advance the measurement of translational science. *J Clin Transl Sci*. 2022 Aug 1;6(1):e107. doi: 10.1017/cts.2022.433. PMID: 36285013; PMCID: PMC9549478. © The Author(s) 2022. This is an Open Access article, distributed under the terms of the Creative Commons Attribution license. (https://creativecommons.org/licenses/by/4.0/. **Reworded.**

Munn Z, Peters MDJ, Stern C, Tufanaru C, McArthur A, Aromataris E. Systematic review or scoping review? Guidance for authors when choosing between a systematic or scoping review approach. *BMC Med Res Methodol*. 2018 Nov 19;18(1):143. doi: 10.1186/s12874-018-0611-x. PMID: 30453902; PMCID: PMC6245623. © The Author(s).2018.CC 4.0. (http://creativecommons.org/publicdomain/zero/1.0/. **Reworded.**

## Chapter 7: Prevention: The Core of Medical Practice

Berben L, Floris G, Wildiers H, Hatse S. Cancer and Aging: Two Tightly Interconnected Biological Processes. *Cancers* (Basel). 2021 Mar 19;13(6):1400. doi: 10.3390/cancers13061400. PMID: 33808654; PMCID: PMC8003441. © 2021 by the authors. Licensee MDPI, Basel, Switzerland. This article is an open access article distributed under the terms and conditions of the Creative Commons Attribution (CC BY) license CC 4.0. Reworded.

https://www.nih.gov/news-events/news-releases/researchers-generate-first-complete-gapless-sequence-human-genome

Wu JW, Yaqub A, Ma Y, Koudstaal W, Hofman A, Ikram MA, Ghanbari M, Goudsmit J. Biological age in healthy elderly predicts aging-related diseases including dementia. *Sci Rep*. 2021 Aug 5;11(1):15929. doi: 10.1038/s41598-021-95425-5. PMID: 34354164; PMCID: PMC8342513. © The Author(s) 2021. **Open Access.** This article is licensed under a Creative Commons Attribution 4.0 International License. To view a copy of this license, **visit** http://creativecommons.org/licenses/by/4.0/. **Reworded.**

Ibid, Wu et al., 2021, reworded.

Bin-Jumah MN, Nadeem MS, Gilani SJ, Al-Abbasi FA, Ullah I, Alzarea SI, Ghoneim MM, Alshehri S, Uddin A, Murtaza BN, Kazmi I. Genes and Longevity of Lifespan. *Int J Mol Sci*. 2022 Jan 28;23(3):1499. doi: 10.3390/ijms23031499. PMID: 35163422; PMCID: PMC8836117. © 2022 by the authors. Licensee MDPI, Basel, Switzerland. This article is an open access article distributed under the terms and conditions of the Creative Commons Attribution (CC BY) license (https://creativecommons.org/licenses/by/4.0/. Reworded.

Poeggeler B, Singh SK, Sambamurti K, Pappolla MA. Nitric Oxide as a Determinant of Human Longevity and Health Span. Int J Mol Sci. 2023 Sep 26;24(19):14533. doi: 10.3390/ijms241914533. PMID: 37833980; PMCID: PMC10572643. © 2023 by the authors. Licensee MDPI, Basel, Switzerland. This article is an open access article distributed under the terms and conditions of the Creative Commons Attribution (CC BY) license (https://creativecommons.org/licenses/by/4.0. Reworded.

Jamil A, Gutlapalli SD, Ali M, Oble MJP, Sonia SN, George S, Shahi SR, Ali Z, Abaza A, Mohammed L. Meditation and Its Mental and Physical Health Benefits in 2023. *Cureus*. 2023 Jun 19;15(6):e40650. doi: 10.7759/cureus.40650. PMID: 37476142; PMCID: PMC10355843. Copyright © 2023, Jamil et al. This is an open access article distributed under the terms of the Creative Commons Attribution License. Reworded.

Montgomery M, Srinivasan A. Epigenetic Gene Regulation by Dietary Compounds in Cancer Prevention. *Adv Nutr*. 2019 Nov 1;10(6):1012-1028. doi: 10.1093/advances/nmz046. PMID: 31100104; PMCID: PMC6855955. Copyright © American Society for Nutrition 2019. This is an Open Access article distributed under the terms of the Creative Commons Attribution License (http://creativecommons.org/licenses/by/4.0. Reworded.

Bure IV, Nemtsova MV, Kuznetsova EB. Histone Modifications and Non-Coding RNAs: Mutual Epigenetic Regulation and Role in Pathogenesis. *Int J Mol Sci*. 2022 May 22;23(10):5801. doi: 10.3390/ijms23105801. PMID: 35628612; PMCID: PMC9146199. © 2022 by the authors. Licensee MDPI, Basel, Switzerland. This article is an open access article distributed under the terms and conditions of the Creative Commons Attribution (CC BY) license. CC 4.0. Quote.

Fang Y, Wang X, Yang D, Lu Y, Wei G, Yu W, Liu X, Zheng Q, Ying J, Hua F. Relieving Cellular Energy Stress in Aging, Neurodegenerative, and Metabolic Diseases, SIRT1 as a Therapeutic and Promising Node. *Front Aging Neurosci*. 2021 Sep 20;13:738686. doi: 10.3389/fnagi.2021.738686. PMID: 34616289; PMCID: PMC8489683. Copyright © 2021 Fang, Wang, Yang, Lu, Wei, Yu, Liu, Zheng, Ying and Hua. This is an open-access article distributed under the terms of the Creative Commons Attribution License (CC BY). Reworded.

Connolly EL, Sim M, Travica N, Marx W, Beasy G, Lynch GS, Bondonno CP, Lewis JR, Hodgson JM, Blekkenhorst LC. Glucosinolates From Cruciferous Vegetables and Their Potential Role in Chronic Disease: Investigating the Preclinical and Clinical Evidence. *Front Pharmacol.* 2021 Oct 26;12:767975. doi: 10.3389/fphar.2021.767975. PMID: 34764875; PMCID: PMC8575925. Copyright © 2021 Connolly, Sim, Travica, Marx, Beasy, Lynch, Bondonno, Lewis, Hodgson and Blekkenhorst. This is an open-access article distributed under the terms of the Creative Commons Attribution License (CC BY). Reworded.

Ağagündüz D, Şahin TÖ, Yılmaz B, Ekenci KD, Duyar Özer Ş, Capasso R. Cruciferous Vegetables and Their Bioactive Metabolites: from Prevention to Novel Therapies of Colorectal Cancer. *Evid Based Complement Alternat Med.* 2022 Apr 11;2022:1534083. doi: 10.1155/2022/1534083. PMID: 35449807; PMCID: PMC9017484. Copyright © 2022 Duygu Ağagündüz et al. This is an open access article distributed under the Creative Commons Attribution License. Reworded.

Rahman MM, Rahaman MS, Islam MR, Rahman F, Mithi FM, Alqahtani T, Almikhlafi MA, Alghamdi SQ, Alruwaili AS, Hossain MS, Ahmed M, Das R, Emran TB, Uddin MS. Role of Phenolic Compounds in Human Disease: Current Knowledge and Future Prospects. *Molecules.* 2021 Dec 30;27(1):233. doi: 10.3390/molecules27010233. PMID: 35011465; PMCID: PMC8746501. © 2021 by the authors. Licensee MDPI, Basel, Switzerland. This article is an open access article distributed under the terms and conditions of the Creative Commons Attribution (CC BY) license (https://creativecommons.org/licenses/by/4.0/. Reworded.

https://dpcpsi.nih.gov/onr/strategic-plan

Sharifi-Rad M, Anil Kumar NV, Zucca P, Varoni EM, Dini L, Panzarini E, Rajkovic J, Tsouh Fokou PV, Azzini E, Peluso I, Prakash Mishra A, Nigam M, El Rayess Y, Beyrouthy ME, Polito L, Iriti M, Martins N, Martorell M, Docea AO, Setzer WN, Calina D, Cho WC, Sharifi-Rad J. Lifestyle, Oxidative Stress, and Antioxidants: Back and Forth in the Pathophysiology of Chronic Diseases. *Front Physiol.* 2020 Jul 2;11:694. doi: 10.3389/fphys.2020.00694. PMID: 32714204; PMCID: PMC7347016. Copyright © 2020 Sharifi-Rad, Anil Kumar, Zucca, Varoni, Dini, Panzarini, Rajkovic, Tsouh Fokou, Azzini, Peluso, Prakash Mishra, Nigam, El Rayess, Beyrouthy, Polito, Iriti, Martins, Martorell, Docea, Setzer, Calina, Cho and Sharifi-Rad. Copyright © 2020 Sharifi-Rad, Anil Kumar, Zucca, Varoni, Dini, Panzarini, Rajkovic, Tsouh Fokou, Azzini, Peluso, Prakash Mishra, Nigam, El Rayess, Beyrouthy, Polito, Iriti, Martins, Martorell, Docea, Setzer, Calina, Cho and Sharifi-Rad. This is an open-access article distributed under the terms of the Creative Commons Attribution License (CC BY). Reworded.

Mohajeri MH. Brain Aging and Gut-Brain Axis. Nutrients. 2019 Feb 18;11(2):424. doi: 10.3390/nu11020424. PMID: 30781628; PMCID: PMC6412679. © 2019 by the author. Licensee MDPI, Basel, Switzerland. This article is an open access article distributed under the terms and conditions of the Creative Commons Attribution (CC BY) license (http://creativecommons.org/licenses/by/4.0. Reworded.

Golovinskaia O, Wang CK. Review of Functional and Pharmacological Activities of Berries. *Molecules*. 2021 Jun 25;26(13):3904. doi: 10.3390/molecules26133904. PMID: 34202412; PMCID: PMC8271923. © 2021 by the authors. Licensee MDPI, Basel, Switzerland. This article is an open access article distributed under the terms and conditions of the Creative Commons Attribution (CC BY) license (https://creativecommons.org/licenses/by/4.0. Reworded.

https://www.fda.gov/consumers/consumer-updates/fda-101-dietary-supplements

Ibid, www.fda.gov

Wang H, Chen W, Li D, Yin X, Zhang X, Olsen N, Zheng SG. Vitamin D and Chronic Diseases. *Aging Dis*. 2017 May 2;8(3):346-353. doi: 10.14336/AD.2016.1021. PMID: 28580189; PMCID: PMC5440113. Copyright: © 2017 Wang, et al. This is an Open Access article distributed under the terms of the Creative Commons Attribution License. Quote.

M Kaźmierczak-Barańska J, Boguszewska K, Karwowski BT. Nutrition Can Help DNA Repair in the Case of Aging. Nutrients. 2020 Nov 1;12(11):3364. doi: 10.3390/nu12113364. PMID: 33139613; PMCID: PMC7692274. © 2020 by the authors. Licensee MDPI, Basel, Switzerland. This article is an open access article distributed under the terms and conditions of the Creative Commons Attribution (CC BY) license (http://creativecommons.org/licenses/by/4.0. Reworded.

https://ods.od.nih.gov/factsheets/list-all

Liu X, Zhang Z, Song Y, Xie H, Dong M. An update on brown adipose tissue and obesity intervention: Function, regulation and therapeutic implications. Front Endocrinol (Lausanne). 2023 Jan 11;13:1065263. doi: 10.3389/fendo.2022.1065263. PMID: 36714578; PMCID: PMC9874101. Copyright © 2023 Liu, Zhang, Song, Xie and Dong. This is an open-access article distributed under the terms of the Creative Commons Attribution License (CC BY). Quote.

Zhu X, Yang J, Zhu W, Yin X, Yang B, Wei Y, Guo X. Combination of Berberine with Resveratrol Improves the Lipid-Lowering Efficacy. *Int J Mol Sci*. 2018 Dec 6;19(12):3903. doi: 10.3390/ijms19123903. PMID: 30563192; PMCID: PMC6321535. © 2018 by the authors. Licensee MDPI, Basel, Switzerland. This article is an open access article distributed under the terms and conditions of the Creative Commons Attribution (CC BY) license (http://creativecommons.org/licenses/by/4.0/. Quote.

Su M, Zhao W, Xu S, Weng J. Resveratrol in Treating Diabetes and Its Cardiovascular Complications: A Review of Its Mechanisms of Action. *Antioxidants* (Basel). 2022 May 30;11(6):1085. doi: 10.3390/antiox11061085. PMID: 35739982; PMCID: PMC9219679 © 2022 by the authors. Licensee MDPI, Basel, Switzerland. This article is an open access article distributed under the terms and conditions of the Creative Commons Attribution (CC BY) license (https://creativecommons.org/licenses/by/4.0. Reworded.

Song YJ, Zhong CB, Wu W. Resveratrol and Diabetic Cardiomyopathy: Focusing on the Protective Signaling Mechanisms. *Oxid Med Cell Longev*. 2020 Mar 13;2020:7051845. doi: 10.1155/2020/7051845. PMID: 32256959; PMCID: PMC7094200. Copyright © 2020 Yan-Jun Song et al. This is an open access article distributed under the Creative Commons Attribution License. Quote.

Gu J, Rao W, Huo S, Fan T, Qiu M, Zhu H, Chen D, Sheng X. MicroRNAs and long non-coding RNAs in cartilage homeostasis and osteoarthritis. *Front Cell Dev Biol*. 2022 Dec 13;10:1092776. doi: 10.3389/fcell.2022.1092776. PMID: 36582467; PMCID: PMC9793335. Copyright © 2022 Gu, Rao, Huo, Fan, Qiu, Zhu, Chen and Sheng. This is an open-access article distributed under the terms of the Creative Commons Attribution License (CC BY). Reworded.

Ghafouri-Fard S, Poulet C, Malaise M, Abak A, Mahmud Hussen B, Taheriazam A, Taheri M, Hallajnejad M. The Emerging Role of Non-Coding RNAs in Osteoarthritis. *Front Immunol*. 2021 Nov 29;12:773171. doi: 10.3389/fimmu.2021.773171. PMID: 34912342; PMCID: PMC8666442. Copyright © 2021 Ghafouri-Fard, Poulet, Malaise, Abak, Mahmud Hussen, Taheriazam, Taheri and Hallajnejad This is an open-access article distributed under the terms of the Creative Commons Attribution License (CC BY). Reworded.

Zhang L, Pitcher LE, Yousefzadeh MJ, Niedernhofer LJ, Robbins PD, Zhu Y. Cellular senescence: a key therapeutic target in aging and diseases. *J Clin Invest*. 2022 Aug 1;132(15):e158450. doi: 10.1172/JCI158450. PMID: 35912854; PMCID: PMC9337830. © 2022 Zhang et al. This work is licensed under the Creative Commons Attribution 4.0 International License. To view a copy of this license, visit http://creativecommons.org/licenses/by/4.0. Reworded.

Xu X, Lai Y, Hua ZC. Apoptosis and apoptotic body: disease message and therapeutic target potentials. *Biosci Rep.* 2019 Jan 18;39(1):BSR20180992. doi: 10.1042/BSR20180992. PMID: 30530866; PMCID: PMC6340950. © 2019. © 2019 The Author(s). This is an open access article published by Portland Press Limited on behalf of the Biochemical Society and distributed under the Creative Commons Attribution License 4.0 (CC BY).

Buoso E, Attanzio A, Biundo F. Cellular Senescence in Age-Related Diseases: Molecular Bases and Therapeutic Interventions. *Cells.* 2022 Jun 26;11(13):2029. doi: 10.3390/cells11132029. PMID: 35805113; PMCID: PMC9266226. © 2022 by the authors. Licensee MDPI, Basel, Switzerland. This article is an open access article distributed under the terms and conditions of the Creative Commons Attribution (CC BY) license (https://creativecommons.org/licenses/by/4.0/.

Faienza F, Rizza S, Giglio P, Filomeni G. TRAP1: A Metabolic Hub Linking Aging Pathophysiology to Mitochondrial *S*-Nitrosylation. *Front Physiol.* 2020 Apr 29;11:340. doi: 10.3389/fphys.2020.00340. PMID: 32411008; PMCID: PMC7201090.Ibid Copyright © 2020 Faienza, Rizza, Giglio and Filomeni. This is an open-access article distributed under the terms of the Creative Commons Attribution License (CC BY). Quote.

Pfeffer CM, Singh ATK. Apoptosis: A Target for Anticancer Therapy. *Int J Mol Sci.* 2018 Feb 2;19(2):448. doi: 10.3390/ijms19020448. PMID: 29393886; PMCID: PMC5855670. © 2018 by the authors. Licensee MDPI, Basel, Switzerland. This article is an open access article distributed under the terms and conditions of the Creative Commons Attribution (CC BY) license (http://creativecommons.org/licenses/by/4.0/. Partial quote.

https://oir.nih.gov/sigs/consciousness-research-interest-group

Thomas S, Jenkins R, Burch T, Calamos Nasir L, Fisher B, Giotaki G, Gnani S, Hertel L, Marks M, Mathers N, Millington-Sanders C, Morris D, Ruprah-Shah B, Stange K, Thomas P, White R, Wright F. Promoting Mental Health and Preventing Mental Illness in General Practice. *London J Prim Care* (Abingdon). 2016 Feb 24;8(1):3-9. doi: 10.1080/17571472.2015.1135659. PMID: 28250821; PMCID: PMC5330334. © 2016 The Author(s). Published by Taylor & Francis. This is an Open Access article distributed under the terms of the Creative Commons Attribution License (http://creativecommons.org/licenses/by/4.0. Reworded.

https://www.un.org/en/development/desa/population/publications/pdf/ageing/WorldPopulationAgeing2019-Highlights.pdf

https://www.census.gov/content/dam/Census/library/publications/2014/demo/p25-1140.pdf (page updated 2021)

Li X, Li Z, Zou Z, Wu X, Gao H, Wang C, Zhou J, Qi F, Zhang M, He J, Qi X, Yan F, Dou S, Zhang H, Tong L, Li Y. Real-Time fMRI Neurofeedback Training Changes Brain Degree Centrality and Improves Sleep in Chronic Insomnia Disorder: A Resting-State fMRI Study. *Front Mol Neurosci*. 2022 Feb 23;15:825286. doi: 10.3389/fnmol.2022.825286. PMID: 35283729; PMCID: PMC8904428. Copyright © 2022 Li, Li, Zou, Wu, Gao, Wang, Zhou, Qi, Zhang, He, Qi, Yan, Dou, Zhang, Tong and Li. This is an open-access article distributed under the terms of the Creative Commons Attribution License (CC BY). Quote.

Ibid, Li et al., 2022, reworded.

https://www.ahrq.gov/questions/resources/going-home/index.html

https://www.cdc.gov/nceh/lead/default.htm

**Chapter 8: Healing Power**

Rosemary the Celtic Lady, Miracles from the Light, Publish America, 2007, first edition.

*Dr.* Joe Dispenza - Creating Miracles with Meditation & The Science of Spontaneous Remissions, June 19, 2022, The Science of Spontaneous Remissions, Heal with Kelly, https://www.youtube.com/watch?v=k4H4yPUqbaw.

Ventegodt S, Merrick J. Clinical holistic medicine: applied consciousness-based medicine. *Scientific World Journal*. 2004 Mar 3;4:96-9. doi: 10.1100/tsw.2004.8. PMID: 15010563; PMCID: PMC5956422. Copyright © 2004 Soren Ventegodt and Joav Merrick. **This is an open access article distributed under the Creative Commons Attribution License. Reworded.**

Rao TS, Asha MR, Jagannatha Rao KS, Vasudevaraju P. The biochemistry of belief. *Indian J Psychiatry*. 2009 Oct-Dec;51(4):239-41. doi: 10.4103/0019-5545.58285. PMID: 20048445; PMCID: PMC2802367. © Indian Journal of Psychiatry. This is an open-access article distributed under the terms of the Creative Commons Attribution License Quote.

**Dr. Larry Dossey - *The Reinvention of Medicine* | *Bioneers*, Dr. Larry Dossey, April 24, 2020. https://www.youtube.com/watch?v=xUsRDxAzn4Y**

Beri K. A future perspective for regenerative medicine: understanding the concept of vibrational medicine. *Future Sci OA*. 2018 Jan 5;4(3):FSO274. doi: 10.4155/fsoa-2017-0097. PMID: 29568563; PMCID: PMC5859346. © 2018 Kavita Beri. This work is licensed under a **Creative Commons Attribution 4.0 License. Quote.**

Syabariyah S, Nurachmah E, Widjojo BD, Prasetyo S, Sanada H, Irianto, Nakagami G, Suriadi, Kardiatun T, Hisan UK. The Effect of Vibration on the Acceleration of Wound Healing of Diabetic Neuropathic Foot Ulcer: A Prospective Experimental Study on Human Patients. *Healthcare* (Basel). 2023 Jan 9;11(2):191. doi: 10.3390/healthcare11020191. PMID: 36673559; PMCID: PMC9859045. 2023 by the authors. Licensee MDPI, Basel, Switzerland. This article is an open access article distributed under the terms and conditions of the Creative Commons Attribution (CC BY) license (https://creativecommons.org/licenses/by/4.0/). Reworded.

Wong RMY, Chow SKH, Tang N, Chung YL, Griffith J, Liu WH, Ng RWK, Tso CY, Cheung WH. Vibration therapy as an intervention for enhancing trochanteric hip fracture healing in elderly patients: a randomized double-blinded, placebo-controlled clinical trial. *Trials.* 2021 Dec 4;22(1):878. doi: 10.1186/s13063-021-05844-y. PMID: 34863272; PMCID: PMC8643183. © The Author(s) 2021. Open Access .This article is licensed under a Creative Commons Attribution 4.0 International License. To view a copy of this licence, visit http://creativecommons.org/licenses/by/4.0/. The Creative Commons Public Domain Dedication waiver (http://creativecommons.org/publicdomain/zero/1.0/. The use of this article cited within this article does not imply endorsement of any article contents, product, or anything else.

Singh A, Varma AR. Whole-Body Vibration Therapy as a Modality for Treatment of Senile and Postmenopausal Osteoporosis: A Review Article. *Cureus.* 2023 Jan 12;15(1):e33690. doi: 10.7759/cureus.33690. PMID: 36793830; PMCID: PMC9925023. Copyright © 2023, Singh et al. This is an open access article distributed under the terms of the Creative Commons Attribution License. Reworded.

Jiang S, Liu H, Li C. Dietary Regulation of Oxidative Stress in Chronic Metabolic Diseases. *Foods.* 2021 Aug 11;10(8):1854. doi: 10.3390/foods10081854. PMID: 34441631; PMCID: PMC8391153. © 2021 by the authors. Licensee MDPI, Basel, Switzerland. This article is an open access article distributed under the terms and conditions of the Creative Commons Attribution (CC BY) license (https://creativecommons.org/licenses/by/4.0/. Reworded.

Kolarovic J, Popovic M, Zlinská J, Trivic S, Vojnovic M. Antioxidant activities of celery and parsley juices in rats treated with doxorubicin. *Molecules.* 2010 Sep 3;15(9):6193-204. doi: 10.3390/molecules15096193. PMID: 20877216; PMCID: PMC6257754. © 2010 by the authors. Licensee MDPI, Basel, Switzerland. This article is an Open Access article distributed under the terms and conditions of the Creative Commons Attribution license (http://creativecommons.org/licenses/by/3.0. Reworded.

Dos Santos Guilherme M, Zevallos VF, Pesi A, Stoye NM, Nguyen VTT, Radyushkin K, Schwiertz A, Schmitt U, Schuppan D, Endres K. Dietary Wheat Amylase Trypsin Inhibitors Impact Alzheimer's Disease Pathology in 5xFAD Model Mice. *Int J Mol Sci*. 2020 Aug 31;21(17):6288. doi: 10.3390/ijms21176288. PMID: 32878020; PMCID: PMC7503408. © 2020 by the authors. Licensee MDPI, Basel, Switzerland. This article is an open access article distributed under the terms and conditions of the Creative Commons Attribution (CC BY) license (http://creativecommons.org/licenses/by/4.0/. Quote.

Di Liberto D, Carlisi D, D'Anneo A, Emanuele S, Giuliano M, De Blasio A, Calvaruso G, Lauricella M. Gluten Free Diet for the Management of Non Celiac Diseases: The Two Sides of the Coin. *Healthcare* (Basel). 2020 Oct 14;8(4):400. doi: 10.3390/healthcare8040400. PMID: 33066519; PMCID: PMC7712796. © 2020 by the authors. Licensee MDPI, Basel, Switzerland. This article is an open access article distributed under the terms and conditions of the Creative Commons Attribution (CC BY) license (http://creativecommons.org/licenses/by/4.0/. Quote.

Roszkowska A, Pawlicka M, Mroczek A, Bałabuszek K, Nieradko-Iwanicka B. Non-Celiac Gluten Sensitivity: A Review. Medicina (Kaunas). 2019 May 28;55(6):222. doi: 10.3390/medicina55060222. PMID: 31142014; PMCID: PMC6630947. © 2019 by the authors. Licensee MDPI, Basel, Switzerland. This article is an open access article distributed under the terms and conditions of the Creative Commons Attribution (CC BY) license (http://creativecommons.org/licenses/by/4.0/. Reworded.

Resveratrol: A Double-Edged Sword in Health Benefits Bahare Salehi, Abhay Prakash Mishra, Manisha Nigam, Bilge Sener, Mehtap Kilic, Mehdi Sharifi-Rad, Patrick Valere Tsouh Fokou, Natália Martins, Javad Sharifi-Rad *Biomedicines*. 2018 Sep; 6(3): 91. Published online 2018 Sep 9. doi: 10.3390/biomedicines6030091 PMCID: PMC6164842 © 2018 by the authors. Licensee MDPI, Basel, Switzerland. This article is an open access article distributed under the terms and conditions of the Creative Commons Attribution (CC BY) license (http://creativecommons.org/licenses/by/4.0/. Reworded.

ACIM, Foundation for Inner Peace, Combined Volume, Third Edition, (ACIM, T-8.IX.1:6-7), p. 158.

https://www.communityservices.act.gov.au/ocyfs/therapeutic-resources/where-is-trauma-stored-in-the-body

De Chiara L, Barcia-Castro L, Gallardo-Gómez M, Páez de la Cadena M, Martínez-Zorzano VS, Rodríguez-Berrocal FJ, Bujanda L, Etxart A, Castells A, Balaguer F, Jover R, Cubiella J, Cordero OJ. Evaluation of Blood Soluble CD26 as a Complementary Biomarker for Colorectal Cancer

Screening Programs. *Cancers* (Basel). 2022 Sep 20;14(19):4563. doi: 10.3390/cancers14194563. PMID: 36230486; PMCID: PMC9559671. © 2022 by the authors. Licensee MDPI, Basel, Switzerland. This article is an open access article distributed under the terms and conditions of the Creative Commons Attribution (CC BY) license (https://creativecommons.org/licenses/by/4.0/. Quote.

Khan MI, Khan MZ, Shin JH, Shin TS, Lee YB, Kim MY, Kim JD. Neuroprotective Effects of Green Tea Seed Isolated Saponin Due to the Amelioration of Tauopathy and Alleviation of Neuroinflammation: A Therapeutic Approach to Alzheimer's Disease. *Molecules*. 2022 Mar 24;27(7):2079. doi: 10.3390/molecules27072079. PMID: 35408478; PMCID: PMC9000224. © 2022 by the authors. Licensee MDPI, Basel, Switzerland. This article is an open access article distributed under the terms and conditions of the Creative Commons Attribution (CC BY) license (https://creativecommons.org/licenses/by/4.0/. Reworded.

Rahmani S, Naraki K, Roohbakhsh A, Hayes AW, Karimi G. The protective effects of rutin on the liver, kidneys, and heart by counteracting organ toxicity caused by synthetic and natural compounds. *Food Sci Nutr*. 2022 Sep 15;11(1):39-56. doi: 10.1002/fsn3.3041. PMID: 36655104; PMCID: PMC9834893. © 2022 The Authors. *Food Science & Nutrition* published by Wiley Periodicals LLC. © 2022 The Authors. *Food Science & Nutrition* published by Wiley Periodicals LLC. This is an open access article under the terms of the http://creativecommons.org/licenses/by/4.0. Quote.

**A Course in Miracles, Foundation for inner Peace, Combined Volume, Third Edition, (T-13.X.6:1-6), p. 263.**

Burnett Heyes S, Pictet A, Mitchell H, Raeder SM, Lau JYF, Holmes EA, Blackwell SE. Mental Imagery-Based Training to Modify Mood and Cognitive Bias in Adolescents: Effects of Valence and Perspective. *Cognit Ther Res*. 2017;41(1):73-88. doi: 10.1007/s10608-016-9795-8. Epub 2016 Aug 8. PMID: 28239214; PMCID: PMC5306169. © The Author(s) 2016

Open Access. This article is distributed under the terms of the Creative Commons Attribution 4.0 International License (http://creativecommons.org/licenses/by/4.0/. Reworded.

Ciborowska P, Michalczuk M, Bień D. The Effect of Music on Livestock: Cattle, Poultry and Pigs. *Animals* (Basel). 2021 Dec 16;11(12):3572. doi: 10.3390/ani11123572. PMID: 34944347; PMCID: PMC8698046. © 2021 by the authors. Licensee MDPI, Basel, Switzerland. This article is an open access article distributed under the terms and conditions of the Creative Commons Attribution (CC BY) license (https://creativecommons.org/licenses/by/4.0. Reworded.

Ibid, Ciborowska et al., 2021, reworded.

Ibid, Ciborowska et al., 2021, reworded.

Matamoros OM, Escobar JJM, Tejeida Padilla R, Lina Reyes I. Neurodynamics of Patients during a Dolphin-Assisted Therapy by Means of a Fractal Intraneural Analysis. *Brain Sci.* 2020 Jun 25;10(6):403. doi: 10.3390/brainsci10060403. PMID: 32630512; PMCID: PMC7349020. © 2020 by the authors. Licensee MDPI, Basel, Switzerland. This article is an open access article distributed under the terms and conditions of the Creative Commons Attribution (CC BY) license (http://creativecommons.org/licenses/by/4.0/. Reworded.

Nair PS, Kuusi T, Ahvenainen M, Philips AK, Järvelä I. Music-performance regulates microRNAs in professional musicians. *PeerJ.* 2019 Mar 29;7:e6660. doi: 10.7717/peerj.6660. PMID: 30956902; PMCID: PMC6442922. © 2019 Nair et al. This is an open access article distributed under the terms of the **Creative Commons Attribution License**. Reworded.

Lestard NR, Capella MA. Exposure to Music Alters Cell Viability and Cell Motility of Human Nonauditory Cells in Culture. *Evid Based Complement Alternat Med.* 2016;2016:6849473. doi: 10.1155/2016/6849473. Epub 2016 Jul 12. PMID: 27478480; PMCID: PMC4960344. Copyright © 2016 N. R. Lestard and M. A. M. Capella. This is an open access article distributed under the Creative Commons Attribution License. Reworded.

www.nccih.nih.gov/health/music-and-health-what-you-need-to-know.

Church D, Stapleton P, Vasudevan A, O'Keefe T. Clinical EFT as an evidence-based practice for the treatment of psychological and physiological conditions: A systematic review. *Front Psychol.* 2022 Nov 10;13:951451. doi: 10.3389/fpsyg.2022.951451. PMID: 36438382; PMCID: PMC9692186. Copyright © 2022 Church, Stapleton, Vasudevan and O'Keefe. This is an open-access article distributed under the terms of the Creative Commons Attribution License (CC BY). Reworded.

The Holy Bible: New King James Version, 1982, Thomas Nelson, **Mark**

Lichtenfeld S, Maier MA, Buechner VL, Fernández Capo M. The Influence of Decisional and Emotional Forgiveness on Attributions. *Front Psychol.* 2019 Jun 25;10:1425. doi: 10.3389/fpsyg.2019.01425. PMID: 31293482; PMCID: PMC6603330. Copyright © 2019 Lichtenfeld, Maier, Buechner and Fernández Capo. This is an open-access article distributed under the terms of the Creative Commons Attribution License (CC BY). Quote.

Akhtar S, Dolan A, Barlow J. Understanding the Relationship Between State Forgiveness and Psychological Wellbeing: A Qualitative Study. *J Relig*

*Health*. 2017 Apr;56(2):450-463. doi: 10.1007/s10943-016-0188-9. PMID: 26932554; PMCID: PMC5320019. © The Author(s) 2016. This article is distributed under the terms of the Creative Commons Attribution 4.0 International License (http://creativecommons.org/licenses/by/4.0/ Reworded.

Rao TS, Asha MR, Jagannatha Rao KS, Vasudevaraju P. The biochemistry of belief. *Indian J Psychiatry*. 2009 Oct-Dec;51(4):239-41. doi: 10.4103/0019-5545.58285. PMID: 20048445; PMCID: PMC2802367. © Indian Journal of Psychiatry/ This is an open-access article distributed under the terms of the Creative Commons Attribution License. Quote.

Enriquez-Geppert S, Smit D, Pimenta MG, Arns M. Neurofeedback as a Treatment Intervention in ADHD: Current Evidence and Practice. *Curr Psychiatry Rep*. 2019 May 28;21(6):46. doi: 10.1007/s11920-019-1021-4. PMID: 31139966; PMCID: PMC6538574. © The Author(s) 2019. This article is distributed under the terms of the Creative Commons Attribution 4.0 International License (http://creativecommons.org/licenses/by/4.0/. Reworded.

A Course in Miracles, Combined Volume Third Edition, Foundation for Inner Peace (T-3.IV.2:3-5) p. 42.

The Holy Bible: New King James Version, 1982, Thomas Nelson, Mark

The Holy Bible: New King James Version, 1982, Thomas Nelson, Philippians

A Course in Miracles (ACIM), Combined volume Third Edition, Foundation for Inner Peace (W-248.1:1-6) Part 11, Lesson 248, p 417.

*Epigenetics, DNA, and PBS* https://www.youtube.com/watch?v=ZcnSfbBmjto&ab_channel=Aferdit aZaja, October 28, 2019.

A Course in Miracles Combined Volume, Third Edition, Foundation for Inner Peace, (T-3.V.2:2-4), p. 44.

A Course in Miracles Combined Volume, Third Edition, Foundation for Inner Peace, T-8.IV.5:4 p. 143.

A Course in Miracles Combined Volume, Third Edition, Foundation for Inner Peace , (ACIM, T-1.I.3:1-3), p 3.

Sobolewska-Nowak J, Wachowska K, Nowak A, Orzechowska A, Szulc A, Płaza O, Gałecki P. Exploring the Heart-Mind Connection: Unraveling the Shared Pathways between Depression and Cardiovascular Diseases. *Biomedicines*. 2023 Jul 5;11(7):1903. doi: 10.3390/biomedicines11071903. PMID: 37509542; PMCID: PMC10377477. © 2023 by the authors.

## Chapter 9: Informing the Future of Healthcare

https://www.nccih.nih.gov/about/nccih-strategic-plan-2021-2025

https://www.nih.gov/about-nih/what-we-do/nih-almanac/national-center-complementary-integrative-health-nccih

Tibboel H, Liefooghe B. Attention for future reward. *Psychol Res.* 2020 Apr;84(3):706-712. doi: 10.1007/s00426-018-1094-4. Epub 2018 Sep 11. PMID: 30206685; PMCID: PMC7109139. © The Author(s) 2018 Open Access. This article is distributed under the terms of the Creative Commons Attribution 4.0 International License (http://creativecommons.org/licenses/by/4.0. Reworded.

Ajmal L, Ajmal S, Ajmal M, Nawaz G. Organ Regeneration Through Stem Cells and Tissue Engineering. *Cureus.* 2023 Jan 29;15(1):e34336. doi: 10.7759/cureus.34336. PMID: 36865965; PMCID: PMC9973391. Copyright © 2023, Ajmal et al. This is an open access article distributed under the terms of the Creative Commons Attribution License. Reworded.

Kozhevnikov M, Elliott J, Shephard J, Gramann K. Neurocognitive and somatic components of temperature increases during g-tummo meditation: legend and reality. *PLoS One.* 2013;8(3):e58244. doi: 10.1371/journal.pone.0058244. Epub 2013 Mar 29. PMID: 23555572; PMCID: PMC3612090. © 2013 Kozhevnikov et al. This is an open-access article distributed under the terms of the Creative Commons Attribution License. Reworded.

Mousavi S. Global Ethical Principles in Healthcare Networks, Including Debates on Euthanasia and Abortion. *Cureus.* 2024 Apr 26;16(4):e59116. doi: 10.7759/cureus.59116. PMID: 38803720; PMCID: PMC11128767. Copyright © 2024, Mousavi et al. This is an open access article distributed under the terms of the Creative Commons Attribution License CC-BY. Quote.

## Chapter 10: Powerful Connections

https://search.earth911

Torres-González OR, Sánchez-Hernández IM, Flores-Soto ME, Chaparro-Huerta V, Soria-Fregozo C, Hernández-García L, Padilla-Camberos E, Flores-Fernández JM. Landfill Leachate from an Urban Solid Waste Storage System Produces Genotoxicity and Cytotoxicity in Pre-Adolescent and Young Adults Rats. *Int J Environ Res Public Health*. 2021 Oct 20;18(21):11029. doi: 10.3390/ijerph182111029. PMID: 34769555; PMCID: PMC8583563. © 2021 by the authors. Licensee MDPI, Basel, Switzerland. This article is an open access article distributed under the terms and conditions of the Creative Commons Attribution (CC BY). Quote.

www.epa.gov/lmop/basic-information-about-landfill-gas#collecting

https://www.epa.gov/landfills/municipal-solid-waste-landfills#:~:text t=Definition,or%20constituents%20from%20those%20wastes.Ammonia https://oceanservice.noaa.gov/facts/eutrophication.htm

Ibid, www.epa.gov

Ibid, www.epa.gov

Prescott SL, Logan AC, Katz DL. Preventive Medicine for Person, Place, and Planet: Revisiting the Concept of High-Level Wellness in the Planetary Health Paradigm. *Int J Environ Res Public Health*. 2019 Jan 16;16(2):238. doi: 10.3390/ijerph16020238. PMID: 30654442; PMCID: PMC6352196. © 2019 by the authors. Licensee MDPI, Basel, Switzerland. © 2019 by the authors. Licensee MDPI, Basel, Switzerland. This article is an open access article distributed under the terms and conditions of the Creative Commons Attribution (CC BY) license (http://creativecommons.org/licenses/by/4.0/.Reworded.

Ibid, Prescott et al., 2019, reworded.

Stewart AG. Mining is bad for health: a voyage of discovery. *Environ Geochem Health*. 2020 Apr;42(4):1153-1165. doi: 10.1007/s10653-019-00367-7. Epub 2019 Jul 9. PMID: 31289975; PMCID: PMC7225204. © The Author(s) 2019. This article is distributed under the terms of the Creative Commons Attribution 4.0 International License (http://creativecommons.org/licenses/by/4.0/. Reworded.

Ibid, Stewart, 2020, reworded.

Hantanasirisakul K, Sawangphruk M. Sustainable Reuse and Recycling of Spent Li-Ion batteries from Electric Vehicles: Chemical, Environmental, and Economical Perspectives. *Glob Chall*. 2023 Jan 26;7(4):2200212. doi: 10.1002/gch2.202200212. PMID: 37020621; PMCID: PMC10069312. © 2023 The Authors. Global Challenges published by Wiley-VCH GmbH. This is an open access article under the terms of the http://creativecommons.org/licenses/by/4.0. Reworded.

Chatterjee J, Dethlefs N. Facilitating a smoother transition to renewable. Energy with AI. *Patterns* (NY). 2022 Jun10;3(6):100528 doi: 10.1016/j.patter.2022.100528. PMID: 35755866; PMCID: PMC9214339.

© 2022 The Author(s) This is an open access article under the CC BY license (http://creativecommons.org/licenses/by/4.0/). Reworded.

https://www.dol.gov/agencies/ilab/reports/child-labor/list-of-goods/supply-chains/lithium-ion-batteries

Ortiz DI, Piche-Ovares M, Romero-Vega LM, Wagman J, Troyo A. The Impact of Deforestation, Urbanization, and Changing Land Use Patterns on the Ecology of Mosquito and Tick-Borne Diseases in Central America. *Insects*. 2021 Dec 23;13(1):20. doi: 10.3390/insects13010020. PMID: 35055864; PMCID: PMC8781098. © 2021 by the authors. Licensee MDPI, Basel, Switzerland. Licensee MDPI, Basel, Switzerland. This article is an open access article distributed under the terms and conditions of the Creative Commons Attribution (CC BY) license (https://creativecommons.org/licenses/by/4.0/. Reworded.

www.stateforesters.org/forest-action-plans

https://www.decadeonrestoration.org/what-ecosystem-restoration.

https://www.un.org/esa/forests

Wang L, Huang D. Nitrogen and phosphorus losses by surface runoff and soil microbial communities in a paddy field with different irrigation and fertilization managements. *PLoS One*. 2021 Jul 9;16(7):e0254227. doi: 10.1371/journal.pone.0254227. PMID: 34242302; PMCID: PMC8274659. © 2021 Wang, Huang. This is an open access article distributed under the terms of the **Creative Commons Attribution License. Reworded.**

Kazmi SSUH, Yapa N, Karunarathna SC, Suwannarach N. Perceived Intensification in Harmful Algal Blooms Is a Wave of Cumulative Threat to the Aquatic Ecosystems. *Biology* (Basel). 2022 Jun 2;11(6):852. doi: 10.3390/biology11060852. PMID: 35741373; PMCID: PMC9220063. © 2022 by the authors. Licensee MDPI, Basel, Switzerland. This article is an open access article distributed under the terms and conditions of the Creative Commons Attribution (CC BY) license (https://creativecommons.org/licenses/by/4.0/. Reworded.

Li W, Chen W, Bian J, Xian J, Zhan L. Impact of Urbanization on Ecosystem Services Balance in the Han River Ecological Economic Belt, China: A Multi-Scale Perspective. *Int J Environ Res Public Health*. 2022 Nov 1;19(21):14304. doi: 10.3390/ijerph192114304. PMID: 36361184; PMCID: PMC9654531. © 2022 by the authors. Licensee MDPI, Basel, Switzerland. This article is an open access article distributed under the terms and conditions of the Creative Commons Attribution (CC BY) license (https://creativecommons.org/licenses/by/4.0/. Reworded.

https://www.epa.gov/saferchoice/learn-about-safer-choice-label

https://www.epa.gov/radon

Prata JC, Silva ALP, da Costa JP, Mouneyrac C, Walker TR, Duarte AC, Rocha-Santos T. Solutions and Integrated Strategies for the Control and Mitigation of Plastic and Microplastic Pollution. *Int J Environ Res Public Health*. 2019 Jul 7;16(13):2411. doi: 10.3390/ijerph16132411. PMID: 31284627; PMCID: PMC6651478. © 2019 by the authors. Licensee MDPI, Basel, Switzerland. This article is an open access article distributed under the terms and conditions of the Creative Commons Attribution (CC BY) license (http://creativecommons.org/licenses/by/4.0/ **Reworded.**

Soong YV, Sobkowicz MJ, Xie D. Recent Advances in Biological Recycling of Polyethylene Terephthalate (PET) Plastic Wastes. *Bioengineering* (Basel). 2022 Feb 27;9(3):98. doi: 10.3390/bioengineering9030098. PMID: 35324787; PMCID: PMC8945055. © 2022 by the authors. This article is an open access article distributed under the terms and conditions of the Creative Commons Attribution (CC BY) license Licensee MDPI, Basel, Switzerland. This article is an open access article distributed under the terms and conditions of the Creative Commons Attribution (CC BY) license (https://creativecommons.org/licenses/by/4.0. **Reworded.**

Ibid, Soong et al., 2022, reworded.

Ullah S, Ahmad S, Guo X, Ullah S, Ullah S, Nabi G, Wanghe K. A review of the endocrine disrupting effects of micro and nano plastic and their associated chemicals in mammals. *Front Endocrinol* (Lausanne). 2023 Jan 16;13:1084236. doi: 10.3389/fendo.2022.1084236. PMID: 36726457; PMCID: PMC9885170. Copyright © 2023 Ullah, Ahmad, Guo, Ullah, Ullah, Nabi and Wanghe This is an open-access article distributed under the terms of the Creative Commons Attribution License (CC BY). Reworded.

Guarnotta V, Amodei R, Frasca F, Aversa A, Giordano C. Impact of Chemical Endocrine Disruptors and Hormone Modulators on the Endocrine System. *Int J Mol Sci*. 2022 May 20;23(10):5710. doi: 10.3390/ijms23105710. PMID: 35628520; PMCID: PMC9145289. © 2022 by the authors. Licensee MDPI, Basel, Switzerland. This article is an open access article distributed under the terms and conditions of the Creative Commons Attribution (CC BY) license CC (https://creativecommons.org/licenses/by/4.0. **Quote.**

Barrett JR. POPs vs. fat: persistent organic pollutant toxicity targets and is modulated by adipose tissue. *Environ Health Perspect*. 2013 Feb;121(2):a61. doi: 10.1289/ehp.121-a61. PMID: 23380189; PMCID: PMC3569705. Reproduced with permission from Environmental Health Perspectives. Reworded.

Lee YM, Jacobs DR Jr, Lee DH. Persistent Organic Pollutants and Type 2 Diabetes: A Critical Review of Review Articles. *Front Endocrinol* (Lausanne). 2018 Nov 27;9:712. doi: 10.3389/fendo.2018.00712. PMID: 30542326; PMCID: PMC6277786. opyright © Lee, Jacobs and Lee. This is an open-access article distributed under the terms of the Creative Commons Attribution License (CC BY). Reworded.

https://www.millenniumassessment.org/en/index.html

https://www.unodc.org/documents/data-and-analysis/wildlife/2020/World_Wildlife_Report_2020_9July.pdf

2017-2020.usaid.gov/sites/default/files/documents/1865/USAID-Report-to-Congress-on-Forestry-and-Biodiversity_FY_2018.pdf

www.unodc.org/documents/data-and-analysis/wildlife/WLC16_Chapter_2.pdf

Ibid, www.unodc.org

Ramamurthy PC, Singh S, Kapoor D, Parihar P, Samuel J, Prasad R, Kumar A, Singh J. Microbial biotechnological approaches: renewable bioprocessing for the future energy systems. *Microb Cell Fact*. 2021 Mar 2;20(1):55. doi: 10.1186/s12934-021-01547-w. PMID: 33653344; PMCID: PMC7923469. © The Author(s) 2021. Open Access. This article is licensed under a Creative Commons Attribution 4.0 International License. To view a copy of this license, visit **http://creativecommons.org/licenses/by/4.0/**. **The Creative Commons Public Domain Dedication waiver (http://creativecommons.org/publicdomain/zero/1.0/. The use of this article cited within this article does not imply endorsement of any article contents, product, or anything else.** Reworded.

www.epa.gov

Pereira RAM, Carvalho NB. Quasioptics for increasing the beam efficiency of wireless power transfer systems. *Sci Rep*. 2022 Dec 3;12(1):20894. doi: 10.1038/s41598-022-25251-w. PMID: 36463379; PMCID: PMC9719471.© The Author(s) 2022. CC 4.0. http://creativecommons.org/licenses/by/4.0/ Quote.

Ibid, Chaterjee & Dethlefs, 2022, reworded.

Hosseini E. Brain-to-brain communication: the possible role of brain electromagnetic fields (As a Potential Hypothesis). *Heliyon*. 2021 Mar 1;7(3):e06363. doi: 10.1016/j.hel7iyon.2021.e06363. PMID: 33732922; PMCID: PMC7937662. © 2021 The Author This is an open access article under the CC BY license (http://creativecommons.org/licenses/by/4.0/). Reworded.

Rao RP, Stocco A, Bryan M, Sarma D, Youngquist TM, Wu J, Prat CS. A direct brain-to-brain interface in humans. *PLoS One*. 2014 Nov 5;9(11):e111332. doi: 10.1371/journal.pone.0111332. PMID: 25372285;Jiang L, Stocco A, Losey DM, Abernethy JA, Prat CS, Rao RPN. BrainNet: A Multi-Person Brain-to-Brain Interface for Direct Collaboration Between Brains. *Sci Rep*. 2019 Apr 16;9(1):6115. doi: 10.1038/s41598-019-41895-7. PMID: 30992474; PMCID: PMC6467884. © 2014 Rao et al. This is an open-access article distributed under the terms of the Creative Commons Attribution License. Reworded.

Jiang L, Stocco A, Losey DM, Abernethy JA, Prat CS, Rao RPN. BrainNet: A Multi-Person Brain-to-Brain Interface for Direct Collaboration Between Brains. Sci Rep. 2019 Apr 16;9(1):6115. doi: 10.1038/s41598-019-41895-7. PMID: 30992474; PMCID: PMC6467884. © The Author(s) 2019. This article is licensed under a Creative Commons Attribution 4.0 To view a copy of this license, visit http://creativecommons.org/licenses/by/4.0/. Reworded.

DeFalco TA, Moeder W, Yoshioka K. Editorial: Ca$^{2+}$ signaling in plant biotic interactions. *Front Plant Sci*. 2023 Jan 20;14:1137001. doi: 10.3389/fpls.2023.1137001. PMID: 36743485; PMCID: PMC9895960. opyright © 2023 DeFalco, Moeder and Yoshioka This is an open-access article distributed under the terms of the Creative Commons Attribution License (CC BY). Reworded.

*Cosmic Ether, Possessing Electric-Tension and Magnetic-Resistance, Is the Unified Field for Physics* Chandrasekhar Roychoudhuri, Physics Department, University of Connecticut, Storrs, USA. *Journal of Modern Physics* > Vol.12 No.5, April 2021. DOI: 10.4236/jmp.2021.125044.

*Physics Lie: There is no Ether,* January 29, 2020. Ray Fleming https://www.youtube.com/watch?v=iNZKwZsF53I&ab_channel=RayFleming

https://www.genome.gov/about-genomics/fact-sheets/Genetics-vs-Genomics, 2018

# About the Author

Darnell Osburn, RN, BSN, is an advocate for licensed practitioners serving medical consumers within the precepts of their healthcare system. Healthcare professionals want to make a difference in the lives of others for various reasons. For me, the magnitude of powerlessness my older sister Barbara and our family experienced during her battle with a chronic illness activated the call to counteract human suffering. This position led to over four decades of clinical care and significant nursing roles that provided a hands-on understanding of the United healthcare delivery system. Each patient encounter has created the space for mutual learning.

As a charge nurse in a psychiatric hospital, my geriatric and then adolescent patients shared their unique stories and struggles. At that time, medicine did not fully understand the degree to which mental health could impact physical health. In some ways, this perception continues. As compassionate care continued in intensive care units and long-term care centers, it was apparent that medical conditions affected emotional and mental well-being. Professional experiences expanded in infection control and prevention, employee health, workers' compensation, and discharge planning. As an RN case manager and utilization review nurse in the insurance industry, clients' needs were assessed.

As a Reiki Master, a different lens and focus heightened my curiosity about energy and the efficacy of various medical systems. This interest launched a ten-year investigative process into the underpinnings of conventional healthcare systems and my role as a nurse healer. Becoming a legal nurse consultant enabled me to identify and analyze gaps between healthcare and the law.

My spouse and I have spent much quality time with family, friends, and our nearly 15-year-old Golden Retriever George (back cover).